THE FLYING VET

THE FLYING VET

AMELIAH SCOTT

WITH DAVID BREWSTER

ABC
BOOKS

Publisher's note: Some of the names of people, places and locations in this book have been changed to protect their privacy.

David Brewster is a Melbourne-based writer whose work is centred on helping memoirists tell their stories. David's published works include *The Nazis Knew My Name*, co-written with Magda Hellinger and Maya Lee, *Scattered Pearls*, co-written with Sohila Zanjani, and *Around the Grounds*, co-written with Peter Newlinds. Visit davidbrewsterwriter.com

The ABC 'Wave' device is a trademark of the Australian Broadcasting Corporation and is used under licence by HarperCollins*Publishers* Australia.

HarperCollins*Publishers*
Australia • Brazil • Canada • France • Germany • Holland • India
Italy • Japan • Mexico • New Zealand • Poland • Spain • Sweden
Switzerland • United Kingdom • United States of America

HarperCollins acknowledges the Traditional Custodians
of the land upon which we live and work, and pays respect
to Elders past and present.

First published in Australia in 2023
by HarperCollins*Publishers* Australia Pty Limited
Gadigal Country
Level 13, 201 Elizabeth Street, Sydney NSW 2000
ABN 36 009 913 517
harpercollins.com.au

A catalogue record for this book is available from the National Library of Australia

ISBN 978 0 7333 4265 3 (paperback)
ISBN 978 1 4607 1554 3 (ebook)

Cover design by Louisa Maggio, HarperCollins Design Studio
Cover images: Kangaroo and cockatoo by shutterstock.com; all other images courtesy of
    author's family archives
Cover photograph by Peter Smith
Author photograph by Brendan Leyden
Typeset in Minion Pro by Kirby Jones
Printed and bound in Australia by McPherson's Printing Group

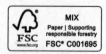

MIX
Paper | Supporting responsible forestry
FSC
www.fsc.org
FSC® C001695

To my supportive family and community. Without you,
I would not have the opportunity to do what I do.

And to my biggest champions – my father and my husband;
I love you both more than I can ever express.

CONTENTS

THE FLYING VET TAKES OFF

I pushed the aeroplane out of the hangar onto the end of our dirt runway, lining it up in the direction of take off. The plane's coat of fresh white paint glistened in the clear morning sun, the green and yellow stripe down the side giving her an extra smart look. I walked around the aircraft, enough hours under my belt by now that I could do my pre-flight checks with confidence. As I dipped the tanks to check the fuel, Dad leaned patiently against the fuselage, his mop of red hair aflame in the golden light. Dad knew his plane like the back of his hand – he flew her nearly every day – but as it wasn't my aircraft, I was always going to take a bit more time.

Finally I climbed into the pilot's seat, while the old man concertinaed his 6 foot 4 (193cm) frame into the passenger's seat. The Cessna 172's cabin is definitely more Mini than Merc. We each pulled our doors closed and donned our headsets. Turning the key, the old gal started instantly, the engine humming smoothly as I did the pre-take off checks known as 'run ups'. I released the brake and pushed the throttle in fully, feeling the plane gather speed as we rolled down the airstrip. As we reached 55 knots, I gently pulled the column towards me. Within seconds we were off the ground.

'I know you haven't started your vet practice yet,' Amanda had said over the phone the day before, 'but I was wondering if you'd be able to come out and see my old pony. She's nearly 35 years old and has lost a lot of weight recently. I think it might be time to say goodbye.'

Amanda was right about my 'practice'. I was a qualified vet by now, with some solid experience under my belt, but I was only home for a brief visit this time. Plans to set up my own business still sat out there in the distance, ever shifting, like the mirage of water on a country road, even if the bush telegraph was already spreading the word.

'I can come tomorrow,' I said. 'Do you have an airstrip?'

Having established that Amanda's place did have somewhere to land – not every property does – I asked her about the condition of the strip. Many airstrips on cattle stations aren't used much and get overgrown or uneven. Getting a wheel caught in a pothole or having the propeller strike the ground during landing or take off would be dangerous or expensive, most likely both. In Amanda's case, she was able to reassure me that their runway was freshly graded and in good nick.

'It's a north-south strip about 800 metres long, with hop-bush scrub at both ends. There's a powerline running parallel about a kilometre to the west.'

Satisfied, I asked Amanda for the coordinates, checked my navigation charts and drew up my flight plan.

It was a perfect morning, with little wind, and early enough in the day that the cool air lent itself to smooth flying. I turned to smile at the old man, reassured at having him in the passenger seat. I don't like borrowing other people's cars, let alone their aeroplanes; having Dad with me made flying his plane a bit easier. On top of that, I was still a novice at bush flying. I'd learnt to fly in northern Victoria, with plenty of landmarks to find my way around, whereas out here in western NSW everything was red from horizon to horizon – especially during a drought. The airstrips were barely distinguishable from the surrounding country, which made them hard to find, and it was difficult to judge distances when landing. But Dad had spent his life flying over country like this. He was always ready with helpful advice, whether or not I asked for it.

After about 40 minutes, we were getting close to Amanda's place, about 80 kilometres east of Wilcannia.

As it turned out, Dad hadn't done much flying over this particular part of the district and didn't know the property we were aiming for, so we navigated based on time, our coordinates and looking out for landmarks. When I reckoned we were getting close, I flicked on the UHF radio.

'Are you on channel there, Amanda?' I said into my headset.

'Hi Ameliah. I can read you clearly,' she replied.

'I'm not sure if we're close to you or not,' I said. 'There are several homesteads I can see coming up.'

'Just a second,' she said. 'Oh wait, yes – yes, I see you!'

'Oh good,' I said.

We flew close to a homestead that I assumed was Amanda's, but couldn't make out an airstrip.

'I'll drive up and down the strip so you can see my dust,' Amanda suggested when I asked for more help.

I flew a wide circuit around the homestead 1000 feet below, but after several minutes I still couldn't see any raised dust.

I called Amanda again. 'When you said you could see me, was I close, or further away than, say, a few kilometres?'

'Oh no, you were close. I could see you clearly,' she replied. 'I'll drive again.'

I felt a sinking feeling in my gut as I did another wide circle in the plane. We were not at the right property. I couldn't see any dust rising anywhere. The question was, exactly where was I relative to her when she thought she'd seen me?

'I could see you out on the horizon on my right,' she responded to my next, slightly more anxious, call.

Hmm. Did that mean east, west, south or north? Right and left don't mean much unless you know which ordinal direction you're facing. When Amanda couldn't answer this question, I turned to share a knowing look with Dad. We couldn't fly around in circles all day. We'd run out of fuel eventually, or not have enough left to fly home. I decided to put my navigational skills to the test.

'Don't worry,' I told Amanda. 'I'll fly to the highway, find your mailbox and follow the drive in from there.'

I turned back towards the north and located the Barrier Highway while Amanda relayed a description of what their main entrance looked like from the road. After following the highway west a short way, I spotted the mailbox and could just make out the sign for the station across the large double gates. I turned south and followed the 12-kilometre driveway to the house, realising that we had only been about 5 kilometres away, quite close after all – though perhaps not as close as it had seemed to Amanda. It was a good lesson for me in the different perspectives of someone on the ground versus someone in the air.

As we neared the house I could clearly see the airstrip to the south, carved into the sandhills with hopbush scrub around it. Dad and I both breathed a sigh of relief. There would be just enough fuel to get us home, plus the mandatory reserve quantity – the amount of fuel the regulators require you to keep spare at all times in case of unforeseen circumstances. I did a quick precursory check of the strip, then set up for landing. I greased the plane down, Dad habitually grabbing for the yoke on his side as we touched down. Do parents ever let go of control?

We were met at the strip by Amanda's father-in-law, a lovely man in his 70s with a jovial face and charming demeanour. He greeted us with warm handshakes. He and Dad had the quick rapport of farmers who have crossed paths at various sales, field days and other social events over many years, even if they lived far enough apart to have never visited each other's properties. Dad and I squeezed into the passenger seat of his Landcruiser ute and he drove us over to the house. He explained that Amanda was over at the stables with her horse, saying what she knew would most likely be her final goodbyes. He offered us the customary cuppa while we waited, him and Dad sharing regional gossip over coffee.

Soon I spotted Amanda walking slowly up to the house, leading the old pony along. The beautiful old horse's head hung low as she made her way beside her owner. I sculled the last mouthful of coffee and left the men to their chat.

It was obvious that Amanda's initial thoughts were right.

'She's had a good life,' I said. 'You've cared for her for a long time. But putting her down is the kindest thing to do now. Let's give her a nice end, rather than having you watch her dwindle even longer.'

A large part of the role of veterinarian is to expose the amount of pain an animal is in. We vets have a moral duty to put the wellbeing of the animal first, even when, as in this case, the kindest and most ethical option is to put an animal to sleep. Sometimes this is because an illness is too far progressed for medical intervention to make a difference, while other times it's because the expenses of potential treatment are clearly beyond the means of the owner.

Sometimes, as with Amanda's pony, euthanasia is just bringing forward the inevitable in order to end the animal's suffering. It can take considerable patience when guiding an owner to this decision, as they grapple with the guilt of not noticing the illness sooner, not being able to afford treatment or simply wanting more time with their beloved pet.

Eventually, most come to accept that euthanasia is the kindest option. The word comes from the Greek, meaning 'good death', which is accurate because it is a painless, fast and kind way of bringing a life to a close. That said, an animal's dying doesn't always look pretty. There are times when chronic pain or the condition an animal has been suffering causes muscle spasms upon loss of consciousness, which can be distressing for owners to have to witness. If I see it coming I encourage owners to look away, or I wrap the pet in a towel so the owner doesn't have this involuntary movement as their last memory of their pet.

'Have you got a nice spot in mind?' I asked Amanda.

'Yes. This morning my husband dug a hole next to a gumtree behind the cattle yards.'

She indicated towards the yards, only 400 metres away.

Giving her shoulder a soft squeeze, I said, 'It will be okay. She'll have a good end. And it looks like a lovely resting place.'

Slowly, in silence, we led the horse over to the chosen site. There is not much you can say in these circumstances. We came to a stop in front of the freshly dug trench. While it sounds macabre, when it comes to euthanising large animals like cows or horses, performing the procedure at the place where they will be buried is the most practical and kindest way for all involved.

Some animals are just too big and heavy to move after they've been put to sleep.

'I'll give her sedation first to keep her calm. Then I'll pop a catheter into her neck vein to administer the final injection,' I explained. 'It's an overdose of anaesthetic, so she won't feel anything while I administer it.'

Amanda nodded in understanding and held the pony still while I sedated her then inserted the catheter. We then led the old pony into the trench.

'This next step will be fast,' I said. 'I'll get you to hold the halter and pat her while I inject the anaesthetic, but once it's all been injected, I'll take her lead rope and you will need to step away. She'll go down in a hurry.'

This is a drawback of putting large animals like horses to sleep. They don't go down gracefully and their weight can be dangerous to vet and owner, adding to the trauma of the situation.

Amanda fondled the pony's forelock as I administered the 'green dream'. I took the rope from her hands as she stepped back, the pony sinking back on her hind quarters then dropping onto her side. It was as good a fall as you could hope for – a 'clean' fall, as my veterinary peers would call it.

Amanda and I stood in silence for a few moments before I confirmed death, checking with my stethoscope that there was no heartbeat. I removed the halter and rope and handed them to Amanda.

'Thank you,' she said, as tears rolled down her cheeks. 'That was the nicest end I've ever seen. All my other old horses have been put down with a bullet, and this is so much kinder.'

I took her arm in mine and steered her towards the house.

'You're welcome,' I said.

A few minutes later Dad and I were back in the plane, Amanda and her father-in-law waving as we took off. An easy, uneventful trip home drew my very first job as a flying vet to a close.

PART ONE

EARLIEST MEMORIES

Flying runs in my blood. I was named after Amelia Earhart, the pioneering aviator who, amongst other achievements, was the first female pilot to fly solo across the Atlantic Ocean. I guess I took that name to heart, because my earliest memories, from when I was probably three or four, are of pestering Dad to join him in the cabin of his plane at every opportunity. From my very first flight, I loved the sensation of being in the sky, completely unattached to anything solid. I still love that feeling as much as ever. Being in the air with Dad felt like total freedom. I loved it when he did a little dip, which made you feel like you were on a roller coaster.

My family has been flying for three generations. My grandfather – my Dad's father – owned and flew a light plane, and both Dad and his sister learnt to fly in their late teens. We fly because it makes sense. Flying is a tool for managing our property and, if necessary, for travelling the long distances between us and any significant signs of civilisation. Where we live in western New South Wales, the distances are vast. The nearest town of White Cliffs has a population of under 200. When we talk about going to 'town', we're referring to Broken Hill, a 540-kilometre round trip away. That's where our nearest supermarket is. There's no ducking around the corner for milk out here!

The family property is one of those outback Australian stations you imagine from books like *We of the Never Never*: wide, flat and dusty under an uninterrupted dome of cobalt sky. We have roughly 60,000 hectares – 150,000 acres in the old measure – of red earth, about 25 kilometres deep and 25 kilometres wide. It's mostly flat country with occasional rocky hills, a mixture of scrub bush and open grasslands. We run cattle, sheep and goats on large tracts of land, where they fend for themselves on the native pasture, the number of animals (and hence the income off the farm) depending on the amount of feed available – less in drought, more after rain. This is flood-plain country, which is glorious to see in a good season, when the grass comes up an iridescent green and stretches for miles, little wildflowers popping out amongst the sand hills. We have to make the most of these seasons when they happen. The memory of the last drought is always fresh, and you're always bracing for the next one. To farm out here is to live forever hoping for the next big rain.

I represent the fifth generation of my family to live here. My great-great grandfather settled on the neighbouring station in the 1880s when the district, on the traditional lands of the Wandjiwalgu and Barundji people, first became inhabited by white men. His family gradually built up their land holdings. His son John, my great-grandfather, took on part ownership of some of this land, then added the rest when a huge sheep station called 'Momba', part-owned by 'Cattle King' Sidney Kidman, was broken up and sold during a drought in the 1920s. There was a scramble to build the homestead in the late 1940s to prevent the government resuming the land as unoccupied. After several years in the hands of haphazard managers, the place was in debt for as much as it was worth.

John offered his daughter, Jan, and her husband Bill Scott – my grandparents – his share in the property if they could pull it out of debt, which they did. When John's original partner died, Jan and Bill went back into debt to buy out his family, and with that the Scotts (and their bank) came to be in possession of this sprawling parcel of land in semi-arid Australia. Weathering that debt, the now-obsolete death taxes, government levies and divorce settlements, the last three generations have each effectively paid for the property twice, but it remains ours.

The property's homestead is a monstrosity. It was built at a time when my great-great grandfather was riding the wool boom, so was designed to accommodate an abundant staff, with workers' quarters separated by a verandah from where the lord and lady lived with their family. The house's cream-coloured brick walls have stood up to the elements and help keep the place cool through our long, hot summers. However, as with all old houses, the upkeep was and is never-ending.

My brother and I were born on the exact same date, two years apart: me first, in December 1989, and James in 1991. At that time, my immediate family lived on another property 150 kilometres south. Dad was effectively managing both properties by then, Granddad being close to retirement, so my father would fly back and forth regularly, even daily at busy times. The nature of the seasons out here means that when there is a job to be done in one place, like mustering or marking lambs, that same job has to be done in the other, and at the same time. I was five years old when Dad formally took over from his father and we all moved back to the main Scott property.

As much as I loved flying, I can't say it was always comfortable. We tended to avoid flying with Granddad, whose acrobatic antics turned my older cousins off the idea of learning to fly at all. But flying with Dad also had its drawbacks.

First, there was the smoke. Dad has always been a chain smoker, and in the days before the dangers of passive smoke were fully appreciated, he would happily fill his plane's little cabin with his exhaled fumes while we sat on the back seat breathing them in. Mix that with avgas fumes from the aircraft's engine, stir it around with a bit of turbulence and turn the heat up to high on a warm day and, well, it wasn't always pretty.

One time, when I was about six, we were flying between the two properties when this recipe came together. Feeling more than a little nauseous, I laid my head down into James's lap. Next thing I knew, my brother's breakfast came up … all through my hair. Needless to say, the rest of that trip was less than pleasant, and both the cabin and I needed a good scrub after we landed. And I had a valuable reminder that James was always more prone to air sickness than I was; so much so that he would never share my enthusiasm for being in the air.

Thankfully I was never put off by that incident, the choking atmosphere or my own experiences of air sickness. All that was trumped by the love of floating in the sky. I was always determined that one day it would be me sitting in the pilot's seat.

Dad remembers one of my earliest close encounters with an animal. One day, when I was about 18 months old, he took me down to the workshop to keep an eye on me while he spent the afternoon mending tyres. Preoccupied with his task, he promptly forgot about me and, like any good toddler enjoying the newfound freedom of being able to walk, I wandered off. When Dad eventually looked up, I was nowhere to be seen in the shed. He looked out across the yard, and felt his heart in his throat when he saw me with one of our horses. Old Smokey, a 16-hand-tall, dark brown ex-racehorse. Most of the time Smokey was a real gentleman, only ever plodding along while being led with a young Ameliah in the saddle. But on this occasion I was testing his patience. What Dad saw was a confused Smokey looking back between his front legs at a little girl using his tail as a swinging rope. I was having a wowser of a time, but Dad realised it would only take one impatient kick from the big horse and I would be a goner.

'Come back, Ameliah,' Dad called in a stage whisper.

I dropped Smokey's tail and made my way back over towards the shed. True to form, Smokey didn't move, let alone kick. He just gave me a bemused look as I waddled away.

As well as planes, we have always had horses. Granddad was horse mad, as were Dad's sisters. My first horse of my own was a hand-me-down pony from my cousins. Suzette, a grey 12-hand pony, was very well trained. She would stop on a dime the minute you fell off, which I did loads of times. Every time, she would wait for me to get back to my feet and back in the saddle before we continued on our merry way. The only problem with this was that Suzette gave me a false sense of security. No other horse I have ever ridden has done anything other than gallop away after turfing me.

Like probably every farm in Australia, we had dogs too. There was always a clear demarcation between the pet dogs and the working dogs, but that didn't mean a pet dog couldn't accompany us while we did work around the place. As is common on farms, as soon as James and I were old enough we were expected to contribute to the never-ending list of chores around the place, including helping with fencing and mustering.

Bogan was an Australian terrier cross, with a wiry brown coat and a mischievous appearance. His elongated body suggested some dachshund ancestry in the mix. He was given to us by Granddad, and named after the river that runs through Nyngan, the town Granddad and Grandma had retired to. Bogan joined all of our adventures as we grew up.

James and I were both driving solo (only on the property of course!) by the time we were eight years old, which meant we could do jobs like bore runs. We have a number of bores around the property, which give access to the precious supply of underground water that is the Great Artesian Basin, providing vital water for sheep and cattle in country that is often devoid of any surface water. We can be very thankful for the existence of the Basin, the world's largest underground water source, which sits under much of northern NSW, South Australia and Queensland. Our place is at the southern end of the Basin, where the water is relatively close to the surface and salt levels are lower than in some places.

These days, solar pumps or windmills bring the water up and into plastic tanks, which then feed adjacent water troughs with float valves to keep them full. Most of the time these troughs are the only source of drinking water available to our stock. The systems are self-contained, but every now and again you need to check that everything is working properly – hence the bore runs.

One of my favourite things to do as a young teenager was a bore run on my own, with Bogan sharing the cabin with me. He was small enough to fit in the gap between the seats and the back wall of the cabin of the Daihatsu ute, his wet nose occasionally poking out and pressing against my arm, jolting me out of my reverie while driving. Otherwise, Bogan would stand with his back feet on the passenger seat and his front feet resting on the dash. Occasionally a ghastly odour would fill the cabin, after which the dog would turn towards me with what I'm convinced was a cheeky grin as I released a string of profanities and rolled down the window to gasp for fresh air.

We always had to be careful not to leave Bogan behind any time he joined us to do some job out in a paddock. He was easy to forget because he spent so much time in his hidey-hole behind the seats, but whenever the vehicle was stationary for any length of time, he would get out of the car to mark his territory and have a sniff about. One day, when retuning from a bore run, I realised he was missing. I retraced my steps and found him under the trough at one of the bores, a wedge-tailed eagle watching him from a nearby tree. If he hadn't been smart enough to take cover, he might have been that bird's meal before I got back to him.

Another of Bogan's quirks was his frequent urge to make love to his pillow, or any 'suitable' object really. He would hump legs, items of clothing, the cat ... the list goes on. Our main station hand, Ticka, once dropped his jumper on the ground while working on the roof of the house, only to look down and see Bogan desecrating it.

'You vile animal. Get off, off, off!' Ticka wailed, to no effect.

Over the years we seemed to collect pets with strange habits. Our ginger cat Hickory loved to share an ice cream with us on a hot summer's day, or to ride on the bonnet of the car as we drove the 12 kilometres to the main gate to collect the mail. He was particularly good at keeping snakes at bay around the house. In dry times, snakes would be attracted to the yard in their search for water. We would often be startled by the discovery of a snake lying across a footpath, finding on closer inspection that it was dead, Hickory's claw marks on the body proving that he'd played the superhero once again.

Ticka's dog Chips, short for Chippendale, was another animal in our lives.

Ticka was a local bloke, born and raised in Broken Hill, who now made his living working on stations in our region. When he wasn't staying on a property, he lived in a dugout – a home created in a man-made cave, providing relief from the heat – in White Cliffs. He spent a lot of time at our place when we were young, helping Dad with the running of the property and making overdue improvements. With deeply tanned skin from years of working outdoors and a cheeky twinkle in his hazel eyes, he always carried a pouch of tobacco and a packet of Tally Ho cigarette papers in his shirt pocket. A rollie sitting in the corner of his mouth was part of his working outfit.

Ticka was quite the character. His name was derived from 'lunatic' – shortened to 'tic', then morphing into 'Ticka' – on the basis of some of his illogical habits. He was a terrible alcoholic most of his life, though up to a certain point it was difficult to tell whether he was drunk or sober. Beyond that point, whoever was employing him at the time would have to send him home to dry out. At the same time, he was always pleasant, and a true gentleman, no matter how inebriated, never swearing in front of women and children.

There was always a copy of *Reader's Digest* on Ticka's bed, so he was a font of knowledge as well as being very witty. He was instrumental in shaping my sense of humour in my formative years. One of his favourite stories was of the morning after a long night at the White Cliffs Hotel. Ticka would tell how he awoke in his car to find the barrel of a gun pointing through the window. Looking across at Chips slumbering on the passenger seat, he realised she would be of no help.

'Don't shoot, don't shoot!' Ticka wailed as he slowly sat up to face his adversary.

As his eyes cleared, he was greeted by a bronze figure standing on the Anzac cenotaph. Turned out Ticka had forgotten that he had parked his car right up next to the memorial.

Our neighbour told of noticing Ticka's red Suzuki ute parked on top of a dam bank one summer afternoon. Going over to investigate, he noticed a pile of empty stubbies in the tray of the ute, then saw Ticka splashing about in the water.

'I'd be careful, it's very deep in there,' he called out to Ticka.

'That's irrelevant to me, my good chap!' came Ticka's gleeful reply. 'I only intend to swim on the top of it.'

Chips went wherever Ticka did. His little red four-wheel drive was Chips's home – specifically the passenger seat that Ticka had to replace regularly every time Chips scratched out the foam stuffing. A black-and-tan kelpie, Chips had a stumpy left foot due to being caught in a rabbit trap. The vet had to remove several bones from the foot, which left her walking on the main pad rather than the toes. When Ticka was at the pub, he would always order a dish of deep-fried potato sticks for his 'lady' which, while she was a working dog, didn't have much effect on her lithe figure. In her life, she did become rotund, as did Ticka after he swapped the booze for soft drinks.

A lifetime of abusing his health eventually caught up with Ticka. He was only 57 when he had a heart attack and died. We were all devastated. While Dad had his moments of impatience with Ticka at times, he was in many ways a part of the family. Our consolation was that Chips came to spend her final years with us. She did as she pleased, sleeping on a bed in the old workshop, occasionally waking up to direct her deep bark at visitors. After she died, I cremated her and spread her ashes on Ticka's grave in the White Cliffs Pioneer and General Cemetery.

Of course, having animals in your life means losing them eventually. Before Chips' death I'd experienced the loss of a number of dearly loved pets, bringing me face to face with the inevitability of death. This lesson was made even harsher on a station like ours, where we all-too-regularly saw livestock suffer and perish through droughts. All of this formed my early motivation to become a veterinarian. I knew I wouldn't be able stop animals dying altogether, but I also knew I would be able give some a longer, happier life, or to at least reduce their suffering. This idea was reinforced by watching Dr Harry Cooper on television, and the care he showed for both animals and their people.

Once I'd settled on this ambition, it wasn't long before my desire to fly found its way in and I started answering the inevitable question of 'What do you want to be when you grow up?' with, 'I'm going to be a flying vet'. What I really meant was that I was going to be a flying vet *at home*, meaning that I would live and operate out of our property. As a kid, the idea of living anywhere else was so foreign to me that it went without saying. Regardless, my response drew a lot of 'That's nice'-type answers from people who either didn't take me seriously or had no idea what I was talking about. They didn't understand how determined this young girl could be.

FAMILY AND PLACE

I n my earliest memory of James, I'm standing up on tippy toes,
peering over the edge of the crib at a sleeping baby. I remember
the jealousy I felt at this new little person taking all the attention
away from me. That was heightened a year later, when I realised
that I would have to share my birthday with him forever!

But as he evolved from baby to toddler to little boy, we
became closer, as much from necessity as anything else. In the
isolation of a remote station, we were each other's everything:
siblings, best friends, school mates, rivals and enemies, all rolled
into one.

Our playground was vast – endless to a child's eye. Like most
kids who grow up on farms, we had the run of the place and would
often disappear for hours, only returning home when hunger
struck. Once we learnt to drive, we could go even further afield.

There were some rules, especially about water. The homestead
sits on the southern side of an almost perfect circle of lake about
one kilometre wide. Fed by a creek that only flows after rain, it
contains water 70 per cent of the time, which is pretty good for

out here. When we were young, swimming without an adult present was a cardinal offence, and even after we learnt to swim we were forbidden from doing so on our own.

This freedom of the wide-open space particularly suited James, a bush kid from the start. When we weren't out adventuring, James was our father's shadow. He was usually seen wearing one of Dad's retired Akubras, the wide brim flopping with every move. He looked like a pocket-sized version of Dad, who was never without an Akubra himself.

When we went into Broken Hill or Sydney, usually to restock or for some sort of appointment, James didn't fully appreciate that things were different in the big smoke. Here, my parents needed to keep vigilant watch on their son, for whenever they let their guard down, he would find something troublesome to occupy himself with.

One time in Sydney we went for dinner at Sizzler, the restaurant every kid loved for its all-you-can-eat dessert bar. The place was packed, but we managed to find a table at the very back. We hadn't even sat down when Dad realised James had absconded. A commotion at the front tables provided a clue, people laughing and pointing. James was discovered with his head under the ice cream dispenser. He had put his mouth under the nozzle and pulled the handle, and after the ice cream came out faster than he could drink it, he let it overflow down the sides of his face, forming messy piles on the floor. By the time Dad got to him, James was covered in the sweet, sticky mess.

On another visit to Sydney, we were taken to see the Christmas display in the Myer front windows, along with a toy 'wonderland' inside. We were wandering through the wonderland when a shop assistant asked if we were missing a little boy. Apparently, there was a child playing in the front display window. To their horror, my parents realised James was indeed missing again. He was found running up and down the large display windows, racing the toy train around its track. With a well-timed grab, Dad caught James by the scruff of his shirt as he ran past, and pulled him out of the display. Once again James had provided some unexpected entertainment to members of the public, while embarrassing his parents no end.

James and I were each other's only primary school classmates since our formal education was provided via a uniquely Australian means: the School of the Air, or SOTA. This meant schooling by a combination of correspondence – mailing materials and assignments back and forth – and classes delivered over two-way shortwave radio. We did our learning this way simply because there was no primary school within a reasonable commuting distance of our property. Our 'school' was based in Broken Hill, nearly 300 kilometres away by road.

The Broken Hill SOTA was originally established in 1956, five years after the world's first School of the Air had been set up in Alice Springs. Both schools, as others in every state of Australia except Tasmania, were made possible by piggy-backing on the radio network that had been set up to support the Royal Flying

Doctor Service. These schools still exist, though the use of paper and two-way radios was gradually replaced by internet-based technologies during the first decade of this century.

With no video link, it was left to our wild imaginings to guess what our teachers and classmates might have looked like. We had a weekly class assembly on a Wednesday morning, with everyone joining in to sing the national anthem. If that creates the impression of a choir of angels over the radio, you'd be wrong. It was definitely cacophony, not choir, each child doing their best to ensure that they stood out amongst the scrambled voices belting out *Advance Australia Fair* over the airwaves.

Many people have the impression that doing schooling via correspondence would provide more flexibility in the timetable. If that happened anywhere it wasn't in our house, where our parents ran our schooling on a schedule of military punctuality. We 'attended' school Monday through Friday from 8 am to 3 pm. There was a half-hour break for morning smoko and an hour for lunch. As there was no risk of passing on disease to the other kids, we had to be at death's door to miss a minute of school. Despite suffering chickenpox, the flu and a debilitating gastric bug at different times, I can count on one hand the number of days I missed of my primary schooling because of sickness. So, no, there was little in the way of extra freedom available to us. The importance of a good education was drilled into us, as was an appreciation for detail and schedules, both of which would hold me in good stead in my pilot training in years to come.

The routine was pretty straightforward. The school would send us a calico library bag of learning materials in the mail once a fortnight. We'd work through it and send our answers back. There was always a bit of overlap, so we never ran out of work. We'd each have a couple of radio lessons a week, and otherwise we were supervised by our governess – our 'govie'. Govies were, and still are, often young women having a gap year between school and university, or between university and a 'real' job. Quite a few have done a teaching degree and use the job to build their confidence before landing in a classroom. (There were also men occasionally, called 'vice teachers', who were often semi-retired teachers looking for a change.)

Govies would stay with us during term, so became part of the family in many ways. If developing classroom skills was their aim, James was only too happy to provide them with practice, always getting up to mischief and being scolded for not paying attention. Truth was, he would have spent every waking moment outside if he could, or if not outside then tinkering in the workshop surrounded by utes, motorbikes and various other farming equipment. He worked out pretty early on that he wanted to be a mechanic when he grew up, so he probably figured he'd learn more by pulling apart motors and putting them back together than he would ever learn from a book. Dad was often left exasperated when he went to use a certain vehicle, only to find its parts strewn across the workshop. On the other hand, I was happy inside, often with my head in a book outside school times.

Doing school by correspondence wasn't completely isolating. Once a year we'd enjoy spending a week with our classmates in Broken Hill, being 'real' school kids for a change. Also at least once a year a teacher from the school would come and visit us for a couple of days. During the year there were various other events where we could see our classmates, like 'mini school', where a group of us would visit a property in the area and stay for a week of activities.

Outside of school, our social lives as children largely revolved around horses, particularly rodeos and gymkhanas. We'd see at least some of our school friends at these events too. Gymkhanas have always been a popular outing for farming families as most children have ponies and many adults keep horses as a recreational pursuit. Because of the travel distances in our part of the world, gymkhanas usually run all weekend and are filled with novelty activities that are really about having fun, for both participants and spectators. Competition is secondary. The children's events are held first, allowing the parents to wear out their children so that, when it comes to having a turn themselves, the kids are too tired to get up to too much strife.

From our point of view, these were weekends when we largely had free rein, at least within the boundaries of the event. We were surrounded by families who all knew each other and kept an eye on each other's children. Events like this were perfect for James, his only problem being that he was always spending any pocket money we were given well before the first day was out. At one gymkhana he became obsessed with the ice cream truck, buying one treat after another. I found James near the end of the day, arguing a case to the vendor that he should be sold a $2.50 ice cream for $2 because that's all he had left. Having hardly spent any of my money, I had to cover that bill. I also had to make sure the rest of my allowance could cover both of us for the rest of the weekend. My strategy with money was, and still is, to never spend a dollar I don't have to. James, clearly more streetwise than me, managed to benefit from my constraint while living it up himself.

One thing I never had exposure to during my primary school years was seeing a real-life veterinarian in practice. In all those years, there was never a vet who serviced our remote region. The closest option for us would have been the clinic in Broken Hill, which was obviously out of the question for large animals or anything urgent.

Secondary school options are extremely limited in the bush, especially when you live as remotely as we did. So, like many kids who grow up on properties, it was off to boarding school for me. I was 11 years old and going into Year 6 when my parents dropped me off at a swanky school in Sydney's eastern suburbs. That day was the first time I saw my dad cry. It was less, I think, because of leaving me there, than due to being overwhelmed by the flood of unpleasant memories of being at boarding school himself.

To say that this move was challenging would be an understatement. It would be for any kid who's spent most of their life living on a remote property, let alone one whose only idea of school life was their little brother and a radio speaker. I had come from an environment of almost entirely men, and now I was sleeping on a bunk bed in a room with seven other girls, eating in a dining room with dozens of others, and going to school with hundreds.

I was wearing a uniform with school shoes and a straw hat and mixing with girls from some of New South Wales's wealthiest families. I'd gone from home, where the closest town of White Cliffs had a population of less than 200, to sharing a city with four million other people. From a place where there were a trillion stars in the night sky, to one where you were lucky to make out the Southern Cross even on a clear evening. From the calls of rosellas, cockatoos and owls to around-the-clock traffic noise.

And to top it all off, I was an obvious target for bullying. Like many pre-teens I was pretty chubby when I started at boarding school, and I clearly didn't fit in to the sort of social aristocracy most others had been brought up in. I was often excluded, called names and teased. Some of the kids enjoyed having a laugh at my expense at bedtime when, unfortunately, some of the mistresses would join in. This went on for three or four years and, looking back now, it's pretty shocking that it was allowed to.

My escape became the library, where I would find a safe spot to hide and read a book. My saviours weren't the teaching staff, but some of the senior girls. A group of nice Year 12s could see what was going on and took pity on me, inviting me to hang out and watch movies with them in their separate boarding house.

It was a pretty lonely time. I didn't really have any friends in those early days, especially in my boarding house. Thankfully I was pretty committed to knuckling down and doing as well as I could with my school work. I was always pretty self-motivated with study, which was fortunate as I'm not naturally smart. I knew I wasn't going to get good grades without hard work. But while I'd love to say I was driven by my dream of becoming a flying vet, that was something for the future. My biggest motivation was to do the best I could as a way of repaying my parents for the enormous financial sacrifices they had made for me. For now, I just had to take advantage of the privilege that had been bestowed on me.

As it turned out, the period when James (who boarded at a school in Bathurst) and I were away at our expensive schools coincided with years of severe drought in western NSW. This, of course, drastically reduced our parents' income, but they were determined that our education wouldn't suffer, and found a way to finance it. There were many visits to the bank over those years, seeking yet another loan. On one occasion all four of us went into the bank after Dad had worded us up on the importance of what he was asking for. I don't know how much it was, but it must have been a fairly big loan given he was more or less putting his children up as collateral!

Eventually the bullying tapered off. I lost weight, which gave them one less thing to pick on me about. I got involved in sport, having a crack at anything, and eventually settling into netball and then touch football when that came on the scene. I was never much good – hand-eye coordination is one thing you don't get much development of in the School of the Air, and unfortunately my city private school offered neither horse riding nor a gun club – but it helped me connect with a few more girls. I also made a few friends, some of whom I'm still very close to today. And I guess I also grew a backbone and started giving it back to the bullies. While I wouldn't recommend copping that sort of treatment as the way to do this, I think what I went through is probably one of the reasons why I don't suffer fools these days.

There weren't a lot of opportunities for flying during my secondary school years. In the best traditions of farming families, our parents would wait until we got home for school holidays before starting the more labour-intensive jobs around the property. That at least gave me the chance to be in Dad's plane with him when there was cattle mustering to be done. We used the plane to provide aerial support to dogs and stockmen on horses as they herded cattle in from the furthest corners of the place, which meant a bit of acrobatic flying at times (and a good test of the old iron stomach).

However, I wasn't able to escape real work by sitting in the aircraft too often. During the height of the drought, what cattle we had were taken to find feed along the road with a drover, often accompanied by Dad. In the summer of 2002, Dad was away doing just that, and it was left to me and James to check the edges of dams and waterholes for sheep that had bogged themselves trying to get a drink. We'd drag them out and, if they were too weak to walk, do the unpleasant job of euthanising them, ideally using a gun. If we didn't have a gun, we had no choice but to use a hard object instead.

Unfortunately, that was the fate of dozens. It was always unpleasant, but also always a better end than the slow death they would have had otherwise. I came across a ewe lambing along the edge of the lake one morning, so we helped her out and away from the boggy mud. Leaving her alone to complete her labour, we went for lunch. On returning, I found she had passed a large lamb, but it was dead and the crows had already pecked its eyes out. To this day, I shudder at the sight of crows.

Despite, or perhaps because of, experiences like this, by the time I got to Year 12 I was still set on becoming a vet. I'd had the chance to do work experience at mixed practice clinics (that is, clinics that serviced both smaller domestic animals and larger animals) in Broken Hill, Young and Longreach and I'd enjoyed it. I was also fairly confident I could get the very high marks I would need to get into veterinary science at university. I knew it was going to take a big effort, but by now I'd proven to myself that I could hack it academically. At the time, the four highest marks in your exams made the most significant contribution to your overall score, so I made a pragmatic decision to let maths, which was compulsory but which I'd struggled with, slip to the bottom of the pile. I put all my effort into everything else, especially English, which I'd always disliked but conquered out of sheer necessity.

I don't remember much about my final exams or receiving the results. What mattered was that I did get a good mark. I ended up receiving offers from a number of the veterinary colleges.

I chose the University of Queensland because of its reputation for a friendly and easy-going attitude, combined with the fact that their vet school had just moved out from the main Brisbane campus to Gatton, a semi-regional location west of Brisbane. With that decided, I felt I was on my way. My feet were planted firmly on the path.

BECOMING A VET

Every young person deserves the chance to go on an adventure and have the freedom to develop into themselves. That is what attending the University of Queensland vet school at Gatton provided me. I was finally studying something I was passionate about, with others who shared that enthusiasm, and I was doing it in a regional location and environment that I was very comfortable with.

One thing that was going to have to wait was learning to fly. It was immediately clear that the university course was going to be demanding of both my brain and my time, and I wasn't going to have much spare money for flying lessons anyway. Instead, I immersed myself into uni life with gusto. There was plenty of study, but it was always balanced by some very serious partying.

The school work in first year combined some basic science with a lot of hands-on work, especially involving dissection of animal cadavers – mainly dogs. That can be pretty grim until you get used to it, but for centuries it's been considered the best way of learning anatomy.

The summer holidays arrived at the end of my first year, in December 2009, and I headed home feeling on top of the world (if you don't count the hangover). One of the benefits of sharing a December birthday with James was that it always fell in the holidays, so we got to celebrate together at home. This year was extra special, as James himself had just finished Year 12 and was looking forward to life after school. From now on we'd be exploring the world as adults, not as kids.

Then, a week after our birthday, my world was shattered.

I don't remember exactly how the day played out. My brain has probably erased the details for my own protection, and there's no point dwelling on them anyway. What I do know is that James was in White Cliffs with three local mates, and that they left town on a dirt road heading north. About a kilometre out of town, their small car left the road. It entered the adjacent table drain and rolled. James and his best mate Mitchell were thrown from the car and killed on the spot; the two kids in the back got away with only minor injuries.

I lost a large part of myself that day. The day, and the weeks that followed, are marred with memories I'd rather I didn't have. The *what-ifs*, *if-onlys* and *what-could-have-beens* struck through my heart; they still do at times.

The rest of that summer holiday is a blur. As the start of my second year approached, I resolved to make the most of my lot and live my life for the person who couldn't. I returned to university without taking any extra time off. It was going to be wrenching, but if I deferred my degree I might never go back.

And so I pushed on, though that year would be by far the hardest of my life, a ceaseless emotional and mental struggle. I wasn't the same person. The joy had gone. Grieving is a complicated process, and my approach was to bury my feelings in study. I was surrounded by others who were filled with optimism about their future, but I could no longer share that feeling. In social situations, I relied on binge drinking, sending myself into an unfeeling oblivion that provided temporary relief. Of course, I always paid the price the morning after.

My parents were struggling with their own demons, and ultimately their marriage folded under the trauma of their grief. Mum moved away. For Dad that meant not only more personal upheaval, but also debt – there was no other way to fund the divorce settlement. It was only a little while later we lost Ticka, making it even more of an *annus horribilus*.

Losing a sibling is the most gut-wrenching tearing apart of your soul. It took a long time, but eventually I was able to remember what had been and relish the precious times we had together, rather than dwell on what would never be. I take comfort in the memories I have of James – of his wit and the way in which he was able to make light of the dullest of circumstances. But the little bugger has forever ruined my birthday. It was bad enough sharing it with him when he was alive.

*

Looking back, I can see that two things got me through that year. The first was the understanding and support I received from a few of my close mates at university. The second was, perhaps unsurprisingly, a dog.

Kay was a young border collie bitch who was left at our place by Dwayne, a contract musterer.

'See if you can get anything out her,' he'd told Dad. 'She's too soft for me.'

After I arrived home for the first semester break, I was soon roped into helping with the job of crutching sheep, the process by which wool is sheared from the crotch and head of the sheep to prevent fly-strike. I'd noticed the shy black-and-white dog sitting in the kennels.

'Can I have her?' I asked Dad.

Having moved off campus into a shared rental house, I had room for a dog in our large backyard.

'If she doesn't do any good over this week, then yes, you can.'

I took the dog with me out in the paddock. She was accustomed to riding on the back of a motorbike, and I enjoyed her soft fur brushing up against my back as she leaned into me. But with the mob of sheep she was timid, weaving back and forth from a distance.

The next day we were crutching again, me picking up the broom as rouseabout. I had the dog with me, and soon she settled herself on a pile of dags (bad, unsaleable wool) in the far corner of the woolshed, where she stayed for the whole day other than a few piddle breaks. She made no attempt to be of any help in the shed whatsoever.

'A completely useless sheepdog,' was one crutcher's description as we pushed the sheep up into the shed without any canine assistance.

It was pretty clear she was not going to cut it as a working dog. Normally this would disappoint me, but on this occasion I was more than happy for her to not show any promise.

So it came to be that she was mine.

Her name was Gay, but that wasn't going to cut it at university. Calling that name around campus could lead to accusations that I was stuck in the '70s. A simple change of the first letter to Kay would solve the problem, so Kay she became. Half her face was white, and half was black; one ear was erect, and the other floppy at the tip. That floppy ear was endearing, flapping rhythmically as she jogged. Her calm personality put me at ease in my darkest hours, her head often resting on my lap in those moments when grief would strike. She would sit with me, leaning against me in a dog-like cuddle as I stroked her, drawing the sadness out of me.

Kay would be my right-hand gal for the next ten years, seeing me though university and the beginning of my veterinary career. I had a responsibility to her to avoid going off the rails. She remained a shy girl, though would instantly warm to anyone who offered food or a pat. She was a good watchdog, to a point. She'd alert the household to any potential intruders into our yard, though I suspect if someone had actually made the effort to breach the boundary, they would have been licked to death.

When I came back from a night out partying in Brisbane, I would be dropped off in the main street of Gatton, then walk down our street. The light posts ended about halfway along, and Kay was always waiting for me there, to escort me through the uncomfortable darkness to the front door.

I did nearly lose her once. While driving back to university after a semester break, I stopped overnight at a friend's house in Moree, about 12 hours into the 18-hour drive. Kay was to sleep under a tree in the back yard. While having dinner, we heard a series of loud popping noises – some kids had lit fire crackers down the street. I ran outside to find that Kay had vanished. Like so many dogs, she was petrified of the noise and had run off in search of refuge. I searched for her that night and again early the next morning, but I couldn't stay to keep looking as I had an exam to get to that afternoon.

Posting lost-dog advertisements with the local newspapers and radio stations was all I could do, aside from just hoping Kay would be found and returned. A very long week later, I had a call from my friend in Moree. She was able to report that, in a situation reminiscent of the movie *Red Dog*, Kay had turned up 100 kilometres north-west of Moree, in Mungindi on the Queensland–New South Wales border. A farmer had been checking his water when he came across a border collie jogging along the roadside. When he pulled over, she'd readily jumped onto the back of his ute, no doubt happy to hitch a ride after all that time on the road.

When I got down there to pick her up, her beautiful soft coat was a tangled, matted mess of burrs. What she had been living on for that week, I'd rather not guess. I had no choice but to shave off her luscious locks, but after a good bath she returned to a more socially acceptable appearance and we resumed our precious partnership.

A year or two after I'd adopted Kay, I was able to return the favour – sort of – to Dad.

I was in the university library with one of my study mates, the two of us diligently doing research like good little students, when Mel told me of her dilemma. Two of her flatmates had taken on a dog together but now, after deciding to move out in different directions, neither wanted to keep the mutt. Mel had no interest in keeping the dog herself either.

'I don't know what to do. I feel sorry for him, but it's going to be hard to find a good home for him because he's hideous!'

I shrugged, thinking she was being overdramatic.

'Show me a picture,' I said.

Mel flicked open her phone and showed me a picture of the dog, who was indeed quite ugly. He was a weedy terrier with a rat-sized body and a wispy, mottled white coat that made him look like he had whiskers around his muzzle. He had a long, pointed nose with a black tip, below small, light brown eyes. His erect ears were too large for his frame.

My heart melted. I've always had a special place there for the ugly ones.

'What's his name?' I asked.

'Dexter,' came the answer, and yes, I could see that in him.

'I have the perfect home for him,' I said.

Since my parents had split up, Dad was home on his own. A bit of furry company in the form of a house-dog would likely help. Our mid-semester break was the following week, so I decided to make the effort and drive home with Dexter. I met Mel to pick up the wiry little mutt, who had so far spent most of his life in an apartment in Brisbane. He was incredibly nervous of people, nervous of anything really, regularly tucking his tail between his back legs and, unhelpfully, piddling himself almost at random.

'He's up-to-date with his vaccinations,' Mel said. 'And here are his toys and bed.' She handed me his lead and placed his few possessions into the back of my car.

I picked the little dog up and popped him onto the front seat, where he didn't move a muscle, as if glued to the upholstery. I had to be very careful with my new passenger on the journey home, and I'm not sure Kay ever really understood what he was about. Dexter seemed constantly petrified of the world. I used several towels on the 18-hour trip, to keep him from ruining my car seats with his nervous incontinence. I started to wonder if it would work out with Dad, but reckoned I'd figure something else out if it didn't.

No sooner had I pulled up and opened the door than Dad was pointing at the hairy, shaking animal on the passenger seat and asking, 'What. Is. That?'

'That,' I said, 'is your new house-yard dog. I thought you could do with a bit of company around here.'

'Hmph, it's a rat!' said Dad. 'What's its name?'

'He was called Dexter by his last owners, but he doesn't respond to that name. I reckon you could rename him if you want to. My housemates thought he looks like a seedy old man and for some reason that made us think of 'Ronald'. Perhaps that might suit?'

So it was that Ronald was inducted into house-yard dog duty at home. His bed, a water bowl and a food bowl were placed underneath the entranceway pergola.

I returned to uni after only a few days, still a bit worried about whether Ronald was going to fit in. My concerns were dispelled the following week when Dad called me.

'That dog you gave me. He's completely bonkers,' he exclaimed. 'I come in the front gate and he runs up to greet me, but he stops about two steps away and rolls onto his back, pissing himself all over and almost getting me with his squirter! Then he gets back up and scampers over for a pat, rolling his piss-soaked foul-smelling little self all over my ankles in the process!'

'He really likes you!' I gushed.

'He followed me halfway across the lawn when I started the pop-up sprinklers the other night. When they came up, he stopped and barked at each one. He couldn't work out how to get through them so he just sat and whined in the middle of the lawn. I had to carry him out. He's completely nuts.'

Initially, Dad thought that, while Ronald was an entertaining addition to the family, he was rather useless. 'A turner,' he called him. 'He turns good tucker into dog shit.'

That changed the day Ronald found his voice. One warm afternoon, Ronald let out a high-pitched bark, and when Dad went to investigate, he discovered a five-foot brown snake making its way towards the house. Turns out Ronald was a bit of a guard dog after all, and from then on he was seen as having some value – enough value to earn a treat any time he barked at intruders, slithering or otherwise.

Unfortunately, in keeping with our family tradition of having crazy pets, Ronald had some other embarrassing habits in his early days of life on the station. He continued to piddle on himself with excitement when you went to pet him, and developed a habit of emptying his bowels in response to a loud noise. Like Bogan before him, he was fond of humping inanimate objects and, unlike Bogan, human legs – especially female legs. This made things rather awkward for Dad after he re-entered the dating world, so I soon had the job of castrating Ronald, which brought that habit to a quick halt.

Perhaps just in time too, for not long after that Dad met Sue, the wonderful lady who would become my stepmother. That came about through a bit of clever matchmaking on the part of me and a local friend of mine who happens to be Sue's daughter. Sue had been working as a station cook in Queensland but was keen to come back closer to Broken Hill, so my friend and I arranged for her to meet Dad. Long story short: it worked!

With the obvious exception of the year after James was taken from us, I enjoyed my time at university. As at school, I needed to work hard, but motivation can take you a long way and I knew this was what I wanted to do.

My graduation at the end of 2013 was a joyous occasion for my family. My aunts, uncles and cousins all came to Gatton to see me receive my Bachelor of Veterinary Science degree with honours. I'm the first doctor of any sort in the family, so that weekend my family members made a big deal of 'being related to the doctor'.

Capitalising on having many hands on deck, we packed up all my goods from the share house, with orders being flung about by various family members. It was getting a bit chaotic when my Uncle Bernie started feeling the pressure of being told what to do by multiple people.

'I'll have you know I'm a doctor's aunty's husband! And I won't be bossed about!' he exclaimed.

Since then our family has replaced the expression 'I'm a monkey's uncle' in our vernacular with 'I'm a doctor's uncle'.

FIRST JOB

With university behind me it was time to get a job. In theory you can qualify as a veterinary surgeon and go straight out and set up your own practice. However, aside from not having the funds I would need to be able to do that, I still had a lot to learn. The best way to go would be to spend a few years in established clinics, gaining experience and learning from seasoned vets.

At the time there was an oversupply of graduates in the market, so I figured I'd strike while the iron was hot. I didn't muck around. In the week immediately after my graduation, instead of driving home, I planned a bit of a tour through NSW and into Victoria, visiting practices that had advertised vacancies on the university's graduate website. I bundled up Kay and Mr Puss, a fluffy cat I'd adopted in my final year, and off we went. I knew I couldn't be too picky given the stiff competition, so I figured I'd focus on finding a nice group of people to work with. Where the job was, and whether they did small animals or large, didn't matter so much. All I had to do was cut my teeth somewhere.

As it turned out, I won the jackpot with my first job. The moment I walked into the clinic in Kerang, in northern Victoria, it felt right. Sarah, one of the senior veterinarians, greeted me in the reception of the small, modern building, and we connected instantly. She showed me around the clinic, with its large windows that allowed plenty of light into both the waiting area and the spacious, open-plan treatment and surgery area at the rear. The whole place was fresh, uncluttered and clean. It didn't have every veterinary toy that you might wish for, but it did have a good vibe.

Working there would also provide me with a wide range of experience. It was a 'mixed practice', meaning they treated both domestic animals and farm animals, and the practice ran two other clinics in the region so there would be geographic variety as well. Sarah's boss, the practice owner, was another vet called Rob, though I didn't meet him that day.

Kerang is a town of around 4000 people that sits on the Loddon River, flowing down from the Murray about 30 kilometres north. This is irrigation country, where water is fed from the rivers into man-made channels that are then used to maintain pasture on adjacent paddocks all year around. This makes for perfect dairy country, and a drive through the area offers scene after scene of black-and-white Friesian and fawn Jersey cows dotted over lush green fields. There are also larger-scale sheep and beef cattle enterprises in the region, as well as broadacre farming of lucerne, canola and other crops. All in all, this was a place where I would be exposed to as wide a range of animals, and clients, as I could have hoped for.

I'd arrived just on smoko, which here meant a pause between morning consults and the day's surgery work. I chatted with the nurse and other associate vet while Sarah made coffees, then helped to ready the surgery patients, putting catheters into their veins and doing pre-anaesthetic examinations. We sipped our coffees while we worked and talked.

I learnt from Sarah that she had emigrated from England 20 years before, and, after doing some work around Australia, she had been whisked off her feet by John Archard, a local dairy farmer. She still retained a strong accent, though her olive skin didn't match the stereotype of the pale Pom. Her short, frizzy blonde hair had the look of being constantly awry, despite her best efforts to contain it.

All of this was my 'interview', and as I felt so much at home so quickly, I had little hesitation in accepting the job offer when it arrived not long after I'd returned home.

Sarah offered to rent me the old cottage on her husband's dairy farm, outside the small town of Murrabit, 30 kilometres north of Kerang. Being out of town and on a property suited me perfectly, and it also meant I could keep Kay and Mr Puss with me. Kay loved the place, with so much room to roam and no shortage of cow dung to roll in. Later I even brought down my horse, Charlie, as the Archards were into horses too and had a good paddock for them. The cottage itself was basic but comfortable, my only fight being against the constant inundation of flies – something for which this region is renowned, and made worse by the cabin sitting right next to the milking shed. The only thing that would keep them at bay inside were automatic fly sprayers, which were fine until the batteries ran out.

Living with the Archards was a bonus in a couple of significant ways.

First, it gave me an instant family, as Sarah, John and their three kids – Becky, 16, Katie, 14, and Will, 11 – were so welcoming. I became a sort of adopted daughter – 'my perfect child' Sarah calls me, though perhaps with a hint of sarcasm because I know I'm far from that. The Archard household was a vibrant, cheerful one in an environment of organised chaos. Three children, a dairy farm and a veterinary career would send most mothers mad, but Sarah managed it all in the Archard's haphazard style. As I left for work, I would often hear her calling out to the children, 'You're going to be late!' as the school bus pulled up at the stop opposite their house. The kids would scramble outside, pulling on uniforms and bags, with pieces of toast hanging from their mouths as they ran.

The second bonus was that I was living on a working farm with 600 Friesian cows that needed looking after, and I had Sarah's vast knowledge to draw on. With so much to learn, the farm became my safe haven, where all mistakes could be forgiven. I made the most of practicing my skills on John's cows and became quite proficient at various surgeries and, in particular, pregnancy testing, a skill cattle farmers need from their vets. The most common form of pregnancy testing for cattle is manual rectal palpitation, which involves slipping your gloved arm into a cow's rectum and feeling for the presence of a foetus in the cervix, which sits under the rectum. This is a quick and cost-effective method that can detect a pregnancy as early as six weeks in. However, it takes a lot of practice. Gaining competence is a numbers game, and this was the perfect place to hone my skill.

John had invested in a lot of modern technology, including a rotary milking platform and computerised milking process. The cows would enter the dairy shed and be milked upon the large, slowly rotating platform while eating their breakfast from feeders on the inside. Whenever I had the chance, usually on a weekend morning, I would set up the treatment platform near the computer screen, then preg-test cows as they drifted past on their giant lazy Susan. I'd cross-check my diagnosis for each animal with the corresponding data entry in John's database. These must have been the most tested cows in the district.

Sarah also taught me a thing or two about maintaining a work-life balance. Once a week, she would have a movie night with her children and I was regularly invited to join in. It was a rare moment in the busy week to enjoy some relaxation.

On one of those nights, John barged into the living room shouting, 'I've got a down cow!'

Without shifting her eyes from the screen, Sarah said, 'Tell a vet who cares.'

I followed her lead, pretending I wasn't there.

She made it quite clear that neither she nor I were vets who cared. It was our night off, and Sarah knew very well that John was a smart enough farmer that he would be able to provide first aid to a fallen cow just as well as we vets would have done.

John borrowed Sarah's keys to pilfer various items from her work car that he would need for the task.

After he left, Sarah looked at me and said, 'Promise me you won't ever marry a dairy farmer.'

It was at the Archard's that I earned an unfortunate nickname.

I involved myself in as many social activities as I could in Murrabit and Kerang, including joining the local netball competition and the adult pony club, but on those weekends when I was on call, I tended to stay on the farm. I took to gardening, discovering that it is one of the few activities that you can leave in the middle of, resuming hours or days later with no major consequences. Over the years I've discovered quite a few vets enjoy gardening precisely for this reason. The Archard children started taking an interest in what I was up to and so, together, we set ourselves the project of building a vegetable patch.

We collected some old corrugated iron water tanks that John had cut down to an appropriate raised-garden-bed height, about mid-thigh level. We laid these out in the bare space behind my cottage, then recruited John to fill them with a mixture of dirt and the abundant manure from the dairy. This garden was never going to be short of compost. Becky directed this earthmoving task, telling her father when each tank was adequately filled, and we then raked out the soil to an even level.

'We could use some mulch on top,' I suggested.

Becky and I both turned and looked at the hay shed, and with knowing nods we headed off in that direction. About halfway over, we walked over a cement block laying in the ground, and as we did so I felt the earth give way underneath me. Before I could do anything, I was falling into the tank. Becky grabbed the collar of my shirt as I fell, but that didn't stop me taking a bath in the tank's foul-smelling, green, soupy water. I soon noticed that I wasn't the only thing bobbing in the liquid either.

'This ... this is the septic tank, isn't it?' I spluttered.

Becky couldn't answer, her mouth clamped shut and nose pinched to block out the smell. She nodded instead.

Great. Just friggin' marvelous, I thought as I hauled myself out of the cesspit. My legs were badly grazed and bleeding from the fall, but most noticeable was the smell of the putrid liquid I was covered in.

Without another word, mulching was cancelled and I squelched back to the cottage. At the back door, I stripped off my clothes and my shoes and threw the lot into the washing machine. I then dived under the shower, scrubbing myself and my injuries several times over to remove the smell and to prevent infection.

We later worked out that the tractor had been driving over the old tank during the veggie bed construction. That had likely cracked the concrete tank's lid, leading to my literal downfall. None of this was my fault, but that didn't stop me becoming 'Dr Poo' to the Archards from that moment on. Before you could say 'septic tank' the story, and my new nickname, had spread around Murrabit as well.

Not long afterwards, just as I was trying to live the nickname down, another unfortunate event sealed the deal.

As a new graduate I was keen to accompany any of the practice vets whenever they attended a more complicated case. Usually I would conduct the initial examination and report my findings, after which we would discuss the case.

One dreary winter's day, I was with my boss, our practice owner, Rob, for a visit to a dairy where the cows had been having trouble with diarrhoea. We needed to conduct a full-scale investigation of the whole herd to ascertain the probable cause. After going over his management of the herd, the farmer told us he had kept one cow aside because she had the worst case of the runs of the lot.

Like a good new grad, I did an extremely thorough clinical exam of this cow. Normally I wouldn't bother with a close inspection of the udder in a case like this, especially if it appears normal. However, this time I was in front of the boss, so I thought I'd better check everything. I reached underneath to inspect the teats closely. As I did so, the cow lifted her tail and expelled the most foul faeces all over me. It went through my hair, ran down my back and found its way into my gumboots.

The men were aghast. I must have looked a dreadful sight. Most people watching a scene like this would have been sent into fits of hysterical laughter, but they just stood with their mouths agape. Once their shock dissipated, they did what they could to help me clean myself with some warm water before I got back into Rob's leather-trimmed Landcruiser Sahara SUV. With the clinic over an hour away, he kindly dropped me at his much closer house to have a shower. I felt like a bedraggled street urchin as his wife guided me into their palatial bathroom.

After that episode, any hope I had that I might be able to escape my new nickname evaporated. The Archards still call me Dr Poo to this day.

EARLY LESSONS

As with most professions, the learning you do at university is only the tip of the iceberg. Your real learning starts when you have to put the theory into practice, and with the complexity of animal care that is inevitably going to mean hard lessons early on. In a practice as busy as Kerang, it also meant that, after a fairly short initial period in which I was supervised by an experienced vet, I was released unchaperoned upon the general public.

For my first solo night on call, I was braced for the worst. I wasn't worried about dealing with emergencies, but instead the opposite. As with all new graduates, I had naïvely thought that after-hours duty would be exciting because I'd be dealing with urgent cases, the more dramatic stuff. I'd soon had those expectations tempered by my colleagues, who told me that about 90 per cent of calls are not emergencies; that instead you get a lot of calls out for a consult that could have waited until opening hours. They also warned me that you get plenty of others simply looking for free advice over the phone because they know they'll get straight through to a vet without having to negotiate their way past a receptionist. On the plus side, I also learnt that, thankfully, being on call didn't mean having to stay awake all night. It just meant keeping the phone by the bed. There are plenty of nights when little happens between midnight and dawn, bar at least a couple of those 'free advice' calls.

On this first night, the on-call gods did their best: they waited until I'd got into my pyjamas before the phone rang. And I was confronted with a genuinely urgent case.

The farmer on the phone had a beef cow with a uterine prolapse. This is a life-or-death condition where the strain of birth has caused the uterus to evert outwards following the birth of the calf. The uterus is literally hanging outside the animal's pelvis, inside-out. Aside from the dangers of having an internal organ outside the body, the uterus is connected to a major vein and artery, and the rupture of either of these could lead to fatal blood loss.

I jumped into the vet car to drive the 50 kilometres north, over the Murray River and along a dark highway to the farm. I left the driveway of the Archard's dairy and turned on my high beam. I used the time I had in the car to plan, step by step, how I was going to tackle the situation. I'd seen and practised prolapses during my university years, so by the time I pulled off the highway I felt that I had a foolproof strategy.

The farmer and his wife waved me over and I pulled up with my headlights directed at the crush holding his cow. A crush is a narrow stall of tubular steel designed to hold an animal still while it gets some sort of examination or treatment. There is typically a 'head bail' at one end, a pair of sliding metal doors that grip the animal just behind the head, and a kick gate at the rear to restrain wayward hooves.

I couldn't have been more unprepared for what greeted me in this crush. Standing in the beam of light was a gigantic Hereford cow. The bottom of her enormous prolapsed uterus was dragging on the ground beneath her. It was, as I would call it later, the mother of all prolapses, to this day the worst I have ever seen. My confidence in my carefully laid plans vanished into the night. I paled as I got my equipment ready, donned my plastic milking apron and squeezed into the crush behind the cow. The meaty, bloody glob of uterus in front was almost as big as I was.

My first step was to administer an epidural as a form of local anaesthetic and to relax her. Without this, the cow would reflexively push against my attempts to manoeuvre the organ back where it belonged. The cow was obese, so I needed to use an extra-long spinal needle to penetrate the thick layer of fat that lay across the top of her tail. Her body wobbled with every move. Nevertheless, I knew my technique had been effective when her tail went limp.

The farmer had several buckets of water at the ready and I used them to give the slimy mass of the uterus a good wash, removing all the dirt and paddock debris it had picked up from the ground. I tucked my apron underneath the bottom of the organ to prevent it from getting dirty again, then went to lift it.

I couldn't. There was no way I was going to be able to pick it up on my own, so I asked the farmer and his wife to each grab a corner of my apron, thus supporting some of the weight of the uterus. I could feel the strain of the mass on my apron's strap as it dug into the back of my neck.

Now I had to get the organ back into the pelvis.

I blocked out the discomfort as, bit by bit, I carefully massaged the slippery, bloody lump of meat back inside. It took force, but I needed to avoid using so much force that I ruptured the tissue. It must have taken an hour – it felt like much longer – to finally heave the last of the uterus up into the pelvis, relieving my neck of the strain. Now I inserted my fist into the vagina and worked to smooth it all back into place. As I was doing this, the cow, sensing the pressure of my fist within her, gave an almighty contraction. It pushed out my arm, closely followed by the entire uterus again. The uterus hit the ground, the light from the car headlights making it clear that I was back to square one. I could have cried in frustration: all that work undone in an instant.

I went back to the car to draw up some muscle relaxant in the hope that it might prevent her from trying to spit the organ out again. Just as I reached the car, I heard a yell behind me. I turned to see that the cow had collapsed, no longer able to hold herself up. She was flailing in the bottom of the crush and risked injuring herself. I got back as the farmer opened the side of the crush to allow her to roll out. She was agonal gasping – gasping for air in a way that indicated she was likely having cardiac arrest. I started cow CPR, which basically involves jumping on the cow's chest – it's much more vigorous than the CPR they teach you in human first aid courses.

The farmer grabbed my arm as I attempted to jump once more after what felt like a thousand compressions. 'You did your best, mate. It's no use,' he said. 'She was in a bad way to start with.'

I stopped and looked down at my patient in the dim light, realising he was right. It had been all bad from the start. She was a huge cow with a huge prolapse. The force of the second prolapse after that contraction would have been enough to rupture the uterine artery, causing death within minutes as it internally bled out faster than a garden hose.

So much for on call being mundane. One night in and I'd managed to deal with a serious emergency and lose my patient at the same time. Still, after facing that calamity, I figured the next time I had to confront a prolapse it would go much more smoothly. How wrong I was. Every vet has a condition that haunts them, and it turned out that the uterine prolapse was to be mine.

Not long after that night, I had to deal with my second prolapse. This one was in daylight, a rare luxury. For whatever reason – perhaps just Murphy's Law – this sort of thing nearly always happens at night. Better still, the family-owned dairy farm was on the edge of Kerang, only about five kilometres from the clinic.

The cow, a Jersey, was quite small, certainly a lot smaller than the Hereford. It was lying down in a green paddock, which was going to make for much easier work than dealing with a standing cow in a dirt-paved yard. I administered the epidural and the farmer and I rolled the cow up onto her sternum, pulling her legs back into a frog-legged position. It was the textbook method in what felt like a textbook situation. I smiled at my progress so far. The uterus was about half my size this time and quite easy to massage back into the pelvis. The farmer was able to stand aside and watch. With everything back inside, I dipped my hand into a bucket of disinfectant and pulled out an empty wine bottle. A wine bottle isn't an official component of the vet's toolkit, but it did work as the perfect extension of my arm to fully revert the uterus back into place within the pelvic cavity. (I'd never got that far with the Hereford.) Satisfied, I stood up, stretching my overworked back as I did so.

The farmer and I manoeuvred the little cow into a more natural sitting position.

'I'll give her some calcium to add some pep to her step,' I said, reaching for a bag of 4-in-1 milk fever injection fluid, cracking the cap off the needle and priming the line, drawing fluid through it to remove any air. The farmer held the cow's head steady with the halter as I located the jugular vein, inserted the needle and began to administer the fluid. *Slowly, slowly,* I reminded myself. The farmer and I were making small talk when I noticed the cow's eyes glaze over. I dropped the fluid pack and jumped onto her chest as I had with the Hereford.

Despite my efforts, I must have given the calcium too quickly, stopping her heart. Once again my attempts at CPR had no effect. She was gone.

I stood there in disbelief. I had done everything by the book. I'd remembered to give the calcium slowly, but obviously not slow enough in this case.

The farmer also looked at the lifeless bovine in disbelief. Thankfully he was an understanding bloke, and after a couple of minutes said, 'I've seen other vets jam that calcium into them with no troubles.'

'She might have had a sensitive heart, but still, it must have been too quick for her,' I replied dejectedly. 'I don't have any other plausible explanation.'

This episode knocked my confidence around, so I approached Rob to ask him for some extra guidance. I was starting to feel that my skills were lagging.

'You've been out in practice for six months,' he said. 'You'll catch up.'

At the same time, he agreed to take me under his wing more often and help me build my skill.

Third time's the charm, or so I've been told. I was on call over the weekend and had just finished playing a game of netball when my phone rang. When the farmer told me it was a prolapse, I groaned inside. Please let me get this one to work, I prayed to the on-call vet gods.

It was an hour's drive away, so I had adequate time to fortify myself. I arrived at the dairy farm mid-afternoon on a pleasant, sunny winter's day. The scene in the paddock wasn't so agreeable. It was not as bad as that first prolapse – again, it was in daylight at least – but the uterus did look a shocking mess. It had been out for some time, judging by the dirt and debris that clung to the drying flesh. I was already wondering if this one might be a little out of my league; whether the tissue may have been past the point of viability and I would need to do an amputation instead to save the animal. It was time to call the big guns.

'Rob,' I said into the phone. 'It looks really bad, and I haven't done a uterine amputation.'

Despite the interruption to weekend activities with his family, Rob readily agreed to come out to help me. Bless him!

It turned out that the uterus wasn't as bad as I'd feared. Once we had given it a thorough cleansing, which took a considerable effort, we removed some of the dead tissue to reveal healthy fresh tissue beneath. Between the two of us, Rob doing most of the work, the uterus popped back into place fairly easily.

I watched diligently as he administered the calcium intravenously, as I had done with the Jersey cow, noting that it seemed to be going in more quickly than I had allowed.

'You've got to go slowly, see?' He showed me how he tipped the bag up and allowed it to run into the vein with minimal assistance, and then every so often he would move the bag so that it was lower than the jugular, stopping the flow of liquid. A backflow of blood coming into the line demonstrated that the needle was still in its correct place within the hose-sized vein along the side of the cow's neck.

He continued administering the entire bag of fluids in this manner until it was all gone. After removing the needle from the neck, Rob went to remove the halter from her head. As he did so, the cow flung herself onto her side, flailing about with her legs stretched.

Rob uttered a bunch of curse words as he sprang into action, jumping up and down on the cow's chest. I heard several of her ribs crack under the greater force he was able to administer. With two of us there we were able to take turns with the CPR but, again, it came to nothing. The animal had gone to cow heaven.

It was late afternoon on a day a few weeks later when I was called out to yet another dairy cow with the cursed predicament. This was another small Jersey, her uterus freshly everted that afternoon after the farmer had finished milking his herd. She was lying down in a nice patch of clean, dry grass and still bright in her demeanour. I rolled my sleeves up and got to work. By now I figured I had nothing to lose, deciding that if the victim of a prolapse was going to die with or without my help, I might as well give it a go.

Finally, everything went by the book. I got the meaty mess up into the pelvis and moulded it into its natural position with relative ease. I gave her the calcium … and she didn't die. *Huzzah!* I administered long-acting antibiotics to fight any infection from dirt that may have been carried back into the pelvic cavity, and explained the aftercare to the farmer.

'I might have to return in a day or two to flush out her uterus,' I said. 'You'll know if this needs to happen – you'll smell it.'

An infected uterus has a stench that clings to the sinuses.

I drove away as the sun set, feeling a profound sense of pride in having completed this task satisfactorily at last.

Several days later, after not hearing from the farmer, I phoned to enquire as to the patient's health.

'She died this morning,' he said.

I put the phone down as my former sense of accomplishment evaporated.

Mother Nature has a way of keeping you on your toes. You'd think that after four bouts of bad luck I would have learnt the limitation of my capabilities, even if one of those had occurred under the hand of a far more experienced vet. Perhaps the successful repair of a prolapse was not on the cards for me. But of course you can't pick and choose the situations you have to deal with.

However, for whatever reason, every prolapse I've attended since this period has gone well, with the uterus easily replaced, the calcium administered, and the cow back on her feet within minutes. And they have all lived to graze another day. What I did to change the winds of fortune, I'll never know. But at least I was able to put that curse behind me.

BUSTED BOOB

It was a lovely spring morning on the Archard's farm. The cows had just finished being milked and were on their wander back to the lush, irrigated pastures nearby, calves calling out as they heard their milk being poured into the 'feeding wagon'. The calves of dairy cows are removed from their mothers immediately after birth, so that the milk the mothers produce can be harvested to start its journey to our supermarkets. The young 'poddy' calves are fed from a wagon, or sometimes by hand, after the herd has been milked, usually on milk from unwell cows that would be unsuitable for human consumption. The feeding wagon is filled from the top and has a heap of teats around the outside that the calves crowd onto.

John had started washing the shed, and I was down at the back of the dairy yard looking at those unwell cows – the so-called 'sick herd'. This group is kept separate from the milking herd to ensure that their milk is treated separately and to prevent the spread of anything contagious.

This was the best assignment I could hope for – literally in my own backyard. On this day my patients included four cows with lame feet, two poor milkers (cows not producing a normal amount of milk) and one dirty cow to flush (I'll get to her).

Of this list, the lame cows were the ones most likely to put a vet into a foul mood. Examination of a cow starts by watching her walk, to understand which leg is afflicted, then guiding her into the crush to make a closer inspection. This inspection involves feeling around the affected limb for swellings or anatomical anomalies. As a vet you are overjoyed if you find the diagnosis at this point; however, that is rarely the case. Most often, you need to tie the foot up, which means wrangling the limb of a 600kg animal up into a safe position so that you can properly inspect the problem hoof – not always easy for a 70kg lady vet. Some smart people have invented gadgets and rope pulleys that make this task a lot easier, but it still isn't pleasant.

A cow's hoof is essentially comprised of two halves, or 'claws', each with its own sole and toe. Often there is a considerable amount of faeces packed around the base of the foot and between the two halves, so you use a hoof knife to clean that out and pare back to the foot itself in search of the inevitable hoof abscess that is the source of the lameness. When you hit the abscess cavity with your knife, watery pus trickles out. Once this is complete, you spray the affected toe with antiseptic, then glue a thin block onto the good toe, which has the effect of elevating the sore side off the ground. The glue used for this is hardcore: it sets within minutes and it sets rock hard. Gloves are imperative, unless you enjoy having your fingers encased in a layer of glue for days afterwards.

None of this is rocket science, and once you've done it a few times it becomes one of the more monotonous and boring tasks of a large animal vet. It's hardly the life-saving surgery you dream of as an aspiring student. After attending to all four lame cows, I was physically drained, but I still had the other three sick cows to look at.

When a cow is 'off her milk', as they call it in the dairy world, it means her milk production has dropped, which is usually because of some sort of illness. These cases are much more interesting for a vet because solving them requires using our brains, flexing our clinical muscles with a series of questions to the herd manager and a thorough clinical exam, before working up the case to a diagnosis. In this case, both the poor milkers were suffering with mastitis, which is easily remedied with some antibiotics and pain relief.

I'd left the 'dirty' cow until last because there was a good chance the work was going to leave me needing a shower. You could smell her from the other side of the dairy yard. Flies congregated in swarms about her vulva. She had calved several days ago, but the placenta had not been expelled and was now rotting, retained within the uterus like uncooked meat forgotten in the fridge. My job was, to put it bluntly, to 'flush out' the uterus, removing the dead material and cleaning up afterwards.

I pulled my rubber milking apron on over my overalls, then donned two pairs of shoulder-length gloves. The hope was that two pairs of gloves would prevent the pungent odour from seeping through into my skin. This effort is always in vain – it's a smell that could permeate bullet-proof steel – but worth a try. I then inserted a tube into the uterine cavity and washed it out with copious amounts of iodine, all while holding my breath and trying my best to ignore the stench.

The cow had sunken eyes, a sure sign of dehydration. I felt for her; it would be miserable to have something rotting inside you for days. I prepared an oral drench of 20 litres of electrolytes, that would be fed via a tube down her throat and directly into her stomach, quickly bolstering her hydration levels. As I lifted her head to introduce the tube, she turned away. Given I'd just removed a gruesome infection from her, I thought she might have been a bit less obstinate, but I guess she wasn't in the mood.

By now my strength was waning from the morning's work, but I only had this simple procedure to finish and I was done. I had to try again. I placed my hand over her muzzle and swung her head up, cradling it into my chest. I was ready to try the tube again, until my hand slipped off her snout. She pulled her head off my chest and turned away, then, with new momentum, she swung her head back towards me, collecting me full on the left side of my chest and instantly knocking the wind out of me. I dropped the drenching equipment, doubling onto my knees on the cement floor of the yard.

Luckily John was still cleaning up and he saw me go down. Racing over to assist, he lifted me back onto my feet, but I couldn't even summon up enough breath to speak to him.

I indicated a stool next to the crush and he helped me take a seat. The pain coursing through my chest was excruciating. I sat there for some time before I finally gasping enough air to groan, 'I'm okay … badly winded.'

John picked up the drenching equipment, finished the job I'd been doing, then released the cow out of the crush. As she walked off towards the paddock, I couldn't help feeling that she glanced back at me as if to say, 'Serves you right.' I was in no position to argue.

'Are you sure you're okay, Dr Poo?' John said with genuine concern. No farmer likes to have one of their animals maiming the vet.

'I'm okay,' I wheezed out. 'I'll have a shower and crack some painkillers. I'll be good as new.'

I hobbled my way towards my cottage.

I was not as good as new. After several brands of painkillers and a cold shower, I could barely dress myself. My entire left side was aching and I couldn't lift my left arm. I'd never realised how imperative the muscles in the chest are to arm movement. I grumbled, frustrated at my lack of mobility. After a bit of a struggle I managed to get my undies on, but there was no way I could get a bra on one-handed. (Why are they so easy to remove one-handed but impossible to get on this way?)

I soon gave up. Today I would need to channel my inner '70s feminist. I pulled on some clean overalls and stuffed my bra and some spare clothes into a plastic shopping bag, then somehow managed to get into the car and drive to work. Luckily it was an automatic. I arrived at the clinic 20 minutes later to find the usual line-up of a dozen small animal patients waiting to see me.

As I worked my way through these consultations, I was constantly aware of my braless state, frequently glancing down to ensure none of the press studs had burst open. In truth I needn't have worried. I am many things, but well-endowed is not one of them.

After getting through the list, I still couldn't raise my left arm, my chest was burning, and my nipples had been rubbed raw inside the thick canvas overalls.

Finally I had time to explain my predicament to the nurse.

'We could wrap your chest with a bandage,' she offered. Then, matter-of-fact, she added, 'You'll need to write up a workplace incident report.'

'What do I write? I've busted my boob?' I said, only half joking.

The reality was, I was embarrassed. It takes a lot to embarrass me, but the thought of someone in the office reading a report about my left boob being squashed by a cow was somehow more than I could bear. Nevertheless, after a fair bit of nagging from the nurse, I eventually typed a report into the computer and sent it off to our practice manager. I was quite chuffed that I'd thought to eloquently describe an injury to my 'mammary tissue' rather than my boob.

Veterinarians are one of those professions in which sick leave is taken as a very last resort, especially when your clinic is as short-staffed as ours was at the time. If you don't work, sick animals won't be seen, so they'll just stay sick. I pressed on, surviving on a cocktail of over-the-counter pain medications, tight chest bandages, and having my arm in a sling. The one reprieve was that I was not on call that week. Or at least, I wasn't meant to be.

A couple of days later, I wasn't much better, when Rob asked me to cover his on-call duties for a short time in the early evening because he was attending a conference. He assured me he'd only be a couple of hours so, as no one else was available, I agreed. I figured my chances of being called out before dark were slim, especially as it was a time of year when dairy cow-related emergencies were unusual.

But Murphy's law struck again. I received a call out to a calving within minutes of taking over the after-hours mobile. The farmer was Bernadette, someone with a reputation for being a 'ball-buster' and from whom I'd been mostly shielded as even the senior veterinarians found her intimidating. The couple of times I had attended her farm, I'd been bombarded with questions as if I was still a student doing practical exams.

'I want Rob to come out,' she said this time, before I got a word in.

'Rob's at a conference tonight. He's asked me to cover, so I'll come straightaway. I have to warn you that I do have an injury due to an accident, so if I can't get the calf out, I'll have to get Rob to come as soon as he's available.'

Not having much choice, Bernadette agreed to this plan. As I drove to her farm, I formulated a plan to assist a calving with one arm. Arriving at the dairy, I pulled up beside the crush, where the brown Jersey-cross cow stood patiently with her head in the bail.

It wasn't until that moment, with only one arm to carry things, that I realised how many buckets I used for a calving. Bernadette took one look at my left arm in a sling and wordlessly came out of the yard and over to the car to help, her renowned gruffness deserting her. Rather than fire a hundred questions off at me as I got started, she helped me ready my equipment and followed my instructions without question.

'Now, I really need two hands to do most of this, but I think with your help we can do it,' I explained, getting her to hold the cow's tail in the correct position as I administered the epidural.

Bernadette poured the obstetrical lubricant over my gloved right arm before I inserted my hand into the vagina, feeling the slimy body of the calf within. It was in the normal presentation except for one tucked-back front leg that was preventing it passing. I reached in further, managing to bring the leg forward and up into the pelvic canal, alongside the head and other front leg.

'I think this will come out relatively well now,' I assured Bernadette. 'I won't be able to pull on the ropes, so if you wouldn't mind doing the hard labour, I'll direct the calf out as you pull.'

She nodded, picking up the rope of the pulley. Sure enough, with only a small amount of effort, the calf slipped out. I unhooked its legs from the calving ropes and we dragged it around to place it in front of the crush so that the cow could lick it all over. The calf opened its eyes for the first time to meet its mum.

Deeply satisfied with my efforts, I cleaned and packed up my gear, Bernadette again helping to carry it for me. Unusually, she stayed to chat while I packed the car. I disguised my surprise and, in no hurry to be anywhere, I took my time, enjoying this moment. Through the conversation I learnt that the real Bernadette wasn't what we saw in the frequently prickly exterior. Probably a bit like myself, if I was honest, she was prone to putting on a tough act. It was a shield to protect her from the judgement of others, as a female farmer operating in a very male world.

It was a valuable lesson to the young me: that a surly demeanour in a client could be more about a level of intimidation than an inherent meanness. My job as a vet was to make my clients feel comfortable around me and to make sure I imparted knowledge in a way that was not condescending.

Other lessons that week included that you can achieve a surprising amount with one arm if you know how to ask for help and work as part of a team. I also learnt that it's important to pay attention and not get so fixated on the job at hand that you leave yourself open to being injured.

Quite the timely education for a youthful and still naïve young vet!

TRICKY SITUATIONS

'I'd like to speak with a *male* vet,' said a deep, insistent voice down the phone.

I drew a deep breath, trying to unclench my jaw. *Who does this bloke think he is?* In a rush of thoughts, I considered launching into a lecture about how 90 per cent of vet graduates are now female, so he'd better get over himself. I also considered using a few four-letter words to tell him where to go. Lucky for him he'd got me on a good day. I opted for the latter approach, but with more tempered language. Well, at least, withholding the expletives.

'Mate, if you can't handle being told what's what by a member of the human race who just happens to have breasts, then you're going to have to search for another vet clinic,' I said. The conversation hadn't started well, and now I was at the end of my tether. 'You'll have to look a long way. If you'd like me to strap on a penis to make you more comfortable accepting the knowledge I'm willing to impart, that can be arranged.'

Clunk was the response as his handset hit the phone.

Good riddance, I thought with satisfaction. I didn't want to deal with a backward-minded insert-four-letter-profanity-here anyway.

I was ten months into being a practicing vet and this was my first experience of real male chauvinism. I was taken aback. Believe it or not, after 25 years on the planet, it was the first time I'd had a man suggest that I couldn't do something because I was a woman.

It wasn't something I'd encountered much in the bush. There is a common misconception that the agricultural sector is more sexist than other industries. It irritates me that one of the first questions I get asked in relation to my career is whether I encounter sexism from farmers. The reality is that farmers are no more sexist than the general population, and perhaps less so. I experience more sexism in town, from people like car dealers, than I do in my work, and my female friends who work in corporate city offices have far more stories to tell than I do. The only times I encounter blatant prejudices like with that caller are in agricultural communities closer to large cities. For some reason, the role of women in many of these communities seems to have remained staunchly traditional for longer, and with that the fossilised views of some men.

In remote farming communities like the one in which I grew up, traditional male–female roles still exist at times, with the mother often caring for young children at home. However, it is not the general opinion any longer that a woman's place is in the kitchen. Farming businesses are true partnerships. It's the only way they can survive. That means the work of both partners is valued, on the land or in the house, no matter who does what. In today's regional communities, women are respected for their ability to do it all.

Back in the days of early white settlement, pioneer women set a high bar for all those who've followed. They often managed the land and raised children on their own while their husbands worked away to make ends meet. Back then, a 4000 hectare (10,000 acre) block was the standard size of a farm across the continent. This was soon revealed to be grossly inadequate to make a living on the drier land of far western New South Wales, so blocks got bigger and the work got harder. Any woman who could cope with living on a property out there in those times was treated like gold, and we still are.

You might be pleased to know that I have other ways of dealing with sexism than by causing men to hang up the phone. Sometimes I can even change a chauvinist's mind.

Mr Gregory was a beef cattle farmer in northern Victoria. Well into his seventies, he was a shortish man with balding head who often wore oversized overalls over a cotton shirt, and a large straw hat. He wouldn't have looked out of place in America's Midwest. He would regularly check his fences on his archaic motorcycle, and had a habit of intently watching any traffic that drove along the road adjacent to his farm. He did this from his house, while standing in a paddock and even while riding his motorbike.

The latter was a bit of a driving hazard. He'd be motoring along, not watching where he was going while his eyes locked on to some known or unknown car on the road. It was comical to witness. I must confess that more than once I deliberately chose to drive along that road for no reason other than the amusement of seeing Mr Gregory stickybeaking while riding his bike.

Not so comical about Mr Gregory was his attitude to female vets. Whenever he called the clinic, he would ask the receptionist to ensure that a male vet would be attending. For a long time they acquiesced, as that was easier than subjecting a female vet to the old grump. But it was not possible to keep going with this approach. At the time I was there the clinic had ten vets, of which only two were male, so it was increasingly unlikely that one of the men could be available at short notice. Instead, the receptionists ended up playing 'Mr Gregory roulette' with us all. They would route the call to all our phones and whoever was unfortunate enough to pick up had to go out there. After a few close shaves, it eventually became my turn.

As with many older farmers on their own, the maintenance of his property had fallen by the wayside. While the fences were suitable for purpose, they were in need of replacement, old barbed wire sagging between lopsided posts. The cattle yards were remnants of a dairy that had been added to over the years, held together with bits of scrap metal and recycled gates.

The first time I went out to his farm was for an outbreak of diarrhoea in his hand-raised calves. The shed in which the calves were housed was an old barn with a dirt floor, small pens along the walls leaving a corridor down the middle. Both ends of the building were open, which created a wind tunnel on a cold winter's day. There were several calves to each pen, and I noted that, while each pen had a clean trough of water, there was not enough hay for them to feed on between mealtimes. The dirt floor and the wind tunnel effect were my main concerns though.

After taking some samples and asking Mr Gregory a few questions about his management practices, I returned to the clinic to run my samples through the laboratory. It didn't take long for me to get a clean-cut diagnosis.

'It's Cryptosporidium – "Crypto" for short,' I explained to him over the phone. In detail I explained how the disease is spread via faeces, and that it could be easily prevented with better hygiene and a few changes to the way he managed his animals.

I got nothing back down the phone. Everything I said seemed to go into one ear and out the other, like his tunnel of a barn.

'I'm not sure I'm understanding you,' he said eventually. 'Could I speak with one of the boys?'

I was sitting in the communal vet's office, with one of 'the boys' sitting right next to me, eavesdropping on my conversation. I rolled my eyes and he returned a smirk.

It took all my patience to be civil.

'Mr Gregory, if you would like a second opinion I can certainly organise another vet to attend. There may be some availability next week.'

So it was that Mr Gregory spent another bundle of money to get a male vet's opinion on his calves, which was exactly the same as mine. I took some consolation from the fact that his sexism had doubled his consulting fees.

Over the coming months I seemed to be allocated to Mr Gregory's more often. I figured it was probably because I had a bit more experience than some of the younger vets in the clinic, and so was more comfortable standing up to him and keeping my cool, at least externally.

But, sure enough, the day came when I finally ran out of patience.

I was attending to yet another calf disease outbreak on Mr Gregory's farm. These calls were common because he would never listen to my advice, or anyone else's, on how to improve his management to prevent his stock getting sick. On this occasion, the weaner-sized steer (about five months old) before me was obviously suffering from neurological deficits, a side-effect of the animal's primary disease, pneumonia. I needed to explain to Mr Gregory the reasons why the calf in front of me was unwell, how the condition could be prevented and how treatment alone would not be sufficient.

'The bacterial infection within his lungs has spread, damaging his brain,' I began.

Looking up at Mr Gregory, I could see he was giving me only scant attention.

'He's fucked in the head,' I said. 'I can make him slightly less fucked with this medication.'

My more abrupt route worked. Mr Gregory's head snapped around and he started nodding vehemently. He didn't break eye contact for the rest of the consultation.

The following week, Mr Gregory rang the clinic. One of the boys answered and said he could come out right away.

'Oh no, not you,' he said. 'Send Ameliah when she's available.'

From that point on I had a great relationship with the old grump and my word was gospel. If only throwing in a few well-articulated profanities could turn every relationship with a sexist client in the same way!

It had been a busy Saturday, but I couldn't switch off completely as I was on call for the weekend. Again. Not unusual for one of the lowest vets in the pecking order. The microwave had no sooner pinged, my quick dinner warmed, than I was called back to the clinic. I looked at the meagre microwave meal with a mixture of disdain and hunger, threw some cling wrap over the top and put it in the fridge. An apple would have to do for now. It would be much easier to chew on the drive.

It was a lovely late spring evening, the canola crops in full golden bloom made even more brilliant by the setting sun. It was almost enough to tempt my eyes away from the road. But with milking just finished, groups of cows meandered down laneways towards lush grazing paddocks, and there was always the chance one or two might stray in front of the car. Most laneways were not fenced in the sturdiest manner, often just a strand of electric tape being all that separated the animals from the highway.

I was going to meet a lady and her sick horse at the clinic. She suspected it had colic, a general term for gut pain. Anything that causes pain in the abdomen will result in colic symptoms, including lack of appetite, pawing at the ground, rolling about, looking at the flank, and reduced defecating, to name a few. It really depends on the cause, and my mind churned though all the possibilities as I approached Kerang.

As I neared the edge of town my phone rang, so I pulled over into a truck bay to answer.

'Are you at the clinic?' said an abrupt female voice. It didn't sound like the lady I had been speaking to earlier.

'Good evening, you have Ameliah,' I said, doing my best to ignore the annoying lack of manners. 'I'm the vet on duty. May I ask who is calling and what can I help you with?'

'I've got a lady in my taxi with her dog. It's really sick, and she wants to go to the vet clinic now.'

There are always a few in the community who assume that a vet lives at the clinic and is ready to serve around the clock. They can get quite irate at the audacity of having to call a vet after hours when they realise the clinic is empty.

'Luckily for your passenger, I'm on my way in to the clinic at the moment. I have another client I'm meeting there.'

We arranged that I would meet the taxi at the front of the clinic. I put the car into gear, checked the mirrors and re-entered the highway.

When I got to the clinic, nobody was there. I unlocked the front door, disabled the alarm and turned on all the lights. There was still plenty of daylight, but it wouldn't last long and I knew little about the cases I was about to deal with.

I was surprised the horse and its owner hadn't arrived yet. Instead, a taxi pulled up in front of the clinic. I went out the front to meet the patient and discovered a woman roughly in her mid-50s, though it was hard to tell as her complexion looked a bit weather beaten. She stood slightly shorter than me as she hunched over a dog in her arms.

The taxi driver drove off almost as soon as her passenger's feet had landed on the ground. I held open the door for my client and followed her inside.

'Good evening,' I said. 'What seems to be the matter with your dog? What's its name?'

When she looked up at me, I took an involuntary step backwards. The woman's face was badly scratched, and her eyes were bloodshot.

'Pup. This is Pup,' she said. 'It's not good.'

With that she began to rock back and forth on her feet, still cradling the dog.

I might have grown up on a remote property, but I hadn't needed to work in Kerang for long before I was exposed to its underside. The town, like so many centres across Australia, struggled with a high incidence of drug addiction, particularly ice (crystal meth). It's a problem that's significantly higher in regional towns than in the major cities, and I'd learnt to read the signs pretty quickly.

I had no doubt the woman standing before me had been using – and given the scabs along her face and on her arms, I thought it was likely her drug of choice was ice. I'd heard that ice users who are coming down off the drug often become extra irritable, taking it out on their skin.

I also knew that ice users could be erratic, and I was alone in the clinic with her. As my mind spun, I outwardly maintained my composure and continued as if everything was normal, while also thinking about safety. The back door of the clinic was still locked, so the only way out was via the front door, which was behind the woman.

'I'll need to print off an admission form before I can start a consult,' I said. 'What name are you under?'

She only gave me her first name, but that was enough to bring up a red flag on the system: *Do not under ANY circumstances allow this person into the clinic. Bad debtor. Violent person.*

I wondered if we might have some relatives listed on the system who could help. It was worth a shot in a small town. As I searched the computer, the woman placed her dog on the ground. He looked a happy little fellow and didn't seem unwell from a distance. He cocked his leg on the corner of the desk and emptied his bladder onto the clean clinic floor, so there was clearly nothing wrong with that end.

'I can't seem to find you on the system,' I lied. 'Do you have any relatives or friends who Pup might be listed under?'

She gave me a number of names, and each time I entered a new one, another red flag popped up. I could feel sweat building above my brow as I wondered whether she was aware of the safe full of narcotics just a couple of metres behind me.

At that moment, a car towing a horse float pulled into the front driveway. I took this distraction as an opportunity, excusing myself and walking past the woman towards the door.

I beckoned her to follow me outside and pointed to a bench on the clinic's front patio. 'I've got to attend to this horse emergency. If you could take a seat out here in the meanwhile, I won't be long.'

She nodded and sat on the bench. The dog followed her outside and proceeded to sniff about the garden bed, his tail wagging happily.

As soon as she was outside, I locked the clinic and met the next client at her driver's door as she emerged from her vehicle.

'G'day Eliza.' In a low voice I briefly explained the situation.

'Should we call the police?' she asked.

'I don't think so. She hasn't acted violently towards me and that might unnecessarily escalate things. I'll attend to her out here, after seeing your horse.'

Eliza opened up the float to allow me to examine her pony. The dainty white miniature horse was calm as I entered the trailer, munching hay out of a hanging net at the front.

'She's calmed down since I called you, but I thought I'd better bring her in just to be sure,' said Eliza.

I nodded as I examined the pony. Her vital signs were all normal.

'From what you described, and given how she seems now, it sounds like she was having a spasmodic episode,' I explained. 'I'll give her some pain relief and a drench of fluids to hydrate her.'

My other patient remained with his owner while I re-opened the clinic door to retrieve what I needed to treat the horse, locking it behind me again. When I returned to the float, Eliza held the halter to steady the pony's head while I administered the pain relief into the jugular vein, then inserted a nasogastric tube. The pony was well behaved. Many miniature horses are spoilt and can be difficult to handle as a result, but Eliza bred hers for children's riding and kept them well disciplined. It made my task a lot easier.

We ensured the pony was restrained appropriately for the journey home before closing the float.

'Here's a spare dose of pain relief in case she needs it in the morning,' I said, passing her a capped syringe. 'If you're not comfortable with intravenous injections, you can inject it into the muscle on the side of her neck.'

I indicated the triangular region where it is safest to inject, along either side of the neck forward of the shoulder and below the mane.

'Will you be okay with her?' Eliza cocked her head towards the other woman.

'I think so, but would you mind being my safety switch? I'll call you when I'm done. If you don't hear from me within 20 minutes, could you send the police to the clinic?'

Eliza agreed. As she pulled away from the clinic, I walked back over to the woman on the bench.

'Are you okay?' I asked her.

She didn't look up, her eyes fixed on the ground in front of her.

I knelt down, out of arm's reach, and repeated the question at eye level.

She turned towards me, rocking vigorously. 'I need an injection. I need needles,' she mumbled.

I nodded but didn't answer. Looking at the dog, I asked, 'Is he okay?'

'Mmmhmm,' she said.

I picked up my phone and called the taxi driver on the number she'd called me from. I wasn't happy that she had left me alone with this woman who clearly was not well.

The taxi driver cheerily answered, 'Good evening.'

'G'day, it's the vet. You better pick this lady up and take her to the hospital,' I said.

Her tone changed in an instant. 'Oh, right. Are you sure? Is the dog okay?'

'The dog is fine, but the lady would like to go to the hospital,' I said.

'I s'pose I'll come.' The driver relented and hung up.

I knelt back down. 'The taxi is coming back. She'll take you to the hospital and see that you are looked after. Okay?'

I stayed with her until the taxi arrived and ensured she was safely inside before I left the clinic, then followed them for a few blocks, making sure the taxi did take her to the hospital.

This situation had been resolved without incident, but that isn't always the case. Unfortunately, violence against workers in health environments is a rising problem around the world. Not long after, a nurse making an after-hours call in the Northern Territory was murdered by a patient. The closeness in time of that situation to my own heightened my awareness of the vulnerability of being on call, alone, especially as a woman.

I have never again either attended a clinic after hours or made a home visit without telling someone I trust exactly where I'm going, who I'm with and how long I expect to be.

MY TINDERELLA

It was a double-dare to join the Tinder dating app. I encouraged a friend from vet school to join with me after we'd both found ourselves recently single. We were both in our first jobs as vets, and finding blokes to date who weren't clients was proving difficult.

We'd set up our profiles with the purpose of attracting nice guys, though the reality seemed to be that these were few and far between. It turned out there were a lot of wankerish sorts on the market, and I was doing a lot of swiping left. One drawback of being a single vet in a country town is that *Farmer Wants a Wife* can translate to *Farmer Wants Free Veterinary Care* in some blokes' minds. Nevertheless, eventually I managed to find a handful of more normal blokes to swipe right on and chat with.

One bloke started to stand out. After a few text messages, Brendan started calling me, giving me hope that his intentions were more serious, and we soon agreed to meet. I remember the date clearly, 5 November 2013, because it was Melbourne Cup Day.

When the day came, I was on call, so I asked him to meet me at our sister clinic in Barham, just over the Murray in New South Wales. I was sitting at the front desk doing some paperwork when I heard the unmistakeable burble of a V8 engine and looked up to see a purple XR8 Ford Falcon pulling up. As the windows of the clinic were mirrored, I could safely perve without him knowing, so as he got out of the car, I was able to take the measure of him.

Brendan was tall, wearing sunnies, a t-shirt and shorts. His brown hair was combed in an odd fashion for a man in his late twenties: to the side like that of a choir boy. I smirked at that. I assumed it was an effort to look neat for our first date. As he locked his car, I took a deep breath. I couldn't hide inside forever, so had better get out there.

I pushed myself up, shut down the computer and opened the front door. We greeted each other with an awkward hug. I didn't want to shake his hand like a mate, but I didn't want to be too familiar with him either.

'I thought we could grab some lunch in this café,' I said, indicating the restaurant next door.

The place was bustling. I'd forgotten about the 'race that stops a nation' so it was busier and louder than I'd anticipated. We shared a pleasant lunch, took a passing interest in the race, then got up to pay. Reaching into my pocket, I realised I'd left my purse inside the vet clinic.

I was mortified. Was he going to think I'd done it on purpose? Or that I 'dined and dashed'?

Brendan chuckled as he watched me fumbling through my pockets. 'I'll get it,' he said with a smile.

To this day, he won't let me live that one down.

We'd no sooner stepped out of the café than I had a call out to an old farmer, Mr Bligh, concerned about one of his labradors. Knowing Mr Bligh, I suspected it wasn't exactly an emergency. He lived on his own on a small farm on the outskirts of town, and his movement was restricted by a combination of his age and use of a wheelchair. His two dogs were his main source of company, and he was prone to being a bit of a hypochondriac about them. Having a vet visit was another source of social connection for the old fella.

'Would you like to come for a drive?' I asked Brendan.

I wasn't ready to end our date just yet, and it had been so noisy in the café that we'd only had a pretty superficial conversation.

On the way out to Mr Bligh's, I learnt a bit about Brendan's background. He was from a dairy farm near the north-central Victorian town of Kyabram – dairy farming and Irish blood run on both sides of the family. He and his three sisters had Catholic upbringings, and he was honest enough to admit that having three sisters meant he had been spoilt, getting away with not many household chores. He helped his dad outside though, driving tractors and milking cows. Brendan was a fitter and turner by trade, who did maintenance work at the SPC canning factory in Shepparton.

When he was younger, he spent a season working on the bores at Alexandria Station, often known as Alexandria Downs, in the Northern Territory: the third-biggest cattle station in Australia. My ears pricked up on hearing this. Without wanting to get ahead of myself, it was good to know that this bloke might have some idea of what it would be like to live on a place like my family's.

That afternoon I gave Brendan a real taste of what a relationship with a vet would be like. As we drove our chat was interrupted by several other non-emergency calls, and each time I had to pull over on the side of the road to answer the phone. It took much longer to get to Mr Bligh's than planned.

Mr Bligh was overjoyed to greet us when we pulled up outside his farmhouse. Back in the day, his garden had been a paradise, but the wheelchair had put paid to that, and it was now overgrown. We had to stoop to avoid the thorny branches dangling down from an arch over the entrance.

'Good to see you, Doctor,' he said, clasping my outstretched hand with both of his. He was wearing his usual old-style flat cap, clean clothes and mismatched socks.

'Same to you. How are the boys?' I said, referring to his dogs.

'Well, Tommy seems to be back to his normal self now. He was sleeping a lot this morning, so it would be good if you could give him a check-up though.'

I gave the old man a smile. This was what I had expected. 'Not a problem at all.'

'You know where they'll be,' he said.

Further up the path I found the yellow labradors lazing on the pavers near the front door. The pair of them were both in perfect health, both young and fit. I patted them as I looked at their gum colour and listened to their chests.

I relayed my findings, or lack thereof, to Mr Bligh, who was relieved that they were going to be okay.

'Can I do anything else for you?' I asked. I knew his carers only came to check on him a couple of times during the week.

'Now that you ask, I don't suppose this tall boyfriend of yours could fix my television for me? There was a bit of wind last night and it's played havoc with the antenna.'

'I'm not sure if I would call him my boyfriend. It's our first date,' I explained awkwardly.

'We shall see about this,' quipped Mr Bligh. 'What are your intentions with the good doctor, young man?'

Brendan coughed. 'I'm not sure yet. But I'll have a look at that antenna for you,' he said, deftly changing the subject.

By the time Brendan climbed onto the roof and repositioned the antenna, Mr Bligh had already formed his opinion of the man.

'Not a bad fella, that one,' he said.

And he was right. Turned out Brendan was a pretty good bloke. I realised early on in our relationship that he was cut from better cloth than most.

The development of our relationship will never be the subject of a romance novel – how often does that happen in real life? But we were comfortable with each other and enjoyed each other's company from the start.

After that initial date we saw each other most weekends, him driving to me or vice versa. I soon discovered, to my satisfaction, that he was very comfortable around animals, even those he didn't have much experience with. At one point I decided to test him by suggesting a horse ride. He could sit on a horse, but that was about the extent of his experience, so the 20-kilometre ride we went on that day really tested his mettle, and his backside. But he did it, showing great patience with his horse, Barbie, a stubborn thing that we borrowed from a friend of mine.

I first met Brendan's family at Christmas at his sister's place in Melbourne, only a month after that first date. He met mine on neutral territory too, at an engagement party in Broken Hill a few months later. His first trip home to our place was the following Christmas, in 2014. That was important, because I had made it clear from early on that if we were going to build our lives together, it was eventually going to mean moving to the property where I'd been raised. That was a non-negotiable.

Brendan got an introduction to flying in light aircraft on that trip, after we'd driven to another property where Dad picked us up in his plane. As we arrived over our place, Dad gave him the grand tour of the property from the air. At one point he pulled the controls back ever-so-subtly to put the plane on a slight incline, then gave me a knowing look before looking over his shoulder at Brendan in the back.

'What kind of intentions do you have for my daughter? She's a good girl,' Dad said.

Before Brendan could answer – or change the subject as he had with Mr Bligh – Dad dipped the yoke forward, which gave us the momentary sensation of falling. At that, Brendan threw his arms in the air, hitting the roof of the plane and knocking off a plastic light fitting in the process. Dad and I were in stitches. Brendan soon got the joke, but he firmly grasped the back of my seat for the rest of the flight.

Thankfully Dad's joke didn't put Brendan off the idea of potentially living at our place down the track.

TAKING TO THE SKY

Sometimes in life, you just need to wait for the stars to align. So it was with my desire to fly.

I may share my name with that famous aviator, and descend from a line of bush pilots, but none of that amounted to anything if I wanted to fly myself. I had to start from scratch as a learner like every other wannabe pilot, and that meant taking expensive and time-consuming flying lessons. Through university I'd been too poor, not to mention too busy, to even think about this. In Kerang, I was at least earning an income, but there wasn't a flight school close enough to make learning to fly realistic even if I had been able to find the time. And my next job hardly allowed me the time to breathe, let alone do anything extracurricular.

After a year in mixed practice in Kerang, an opportunity came up to take on an internship at a specialist equine hospital. In a moment of madness – at least in hindsight – I decided to apply for it. I love horses, and these were highly sought-after positions at the time. I figured it would broaden my experience still further.

The level and type of care would be quite different to what I'd experienced around Kerang.

Horses are very valuable animals, which means the level of care they receive can be a lot higher than what is meted out to your average cow. And having had a good relationship with horses since swinging on Smokey's tail as a toddler, I figured working with them would be interesting and rewarding.

I got the job, and once it came time to start, in early 2014, Kay, Mr Puss and I said goodbye and a big thank you to the Archards and headed south, further into Victoria. We moved into a furnished unit in the central Victorian town that was home to the hospital. Mr Puss immediately made his mark, and nearly caused me to become homeless, by disgracing himself on a suede lounge my landlord had only just purchased. Mercifully, the landlord had a soft spot for felines and, understanding their nature, she forgave him for leaving a pile of warm mousse-consistency poop upon the upholstery.

Kay lasted a few months of living in town before I ended up sending her to Brendan's family's farm. As she'd done back in Gatton, she started coming out onto the road to wait for me when I went out for a night call; only this highway was a lot busier than the suburban street had been in rural Queensland. I lived in fear that I would come home one night and find her squished on the road. She was much happier, and safer, once she'd moved back to a farm, where she could be a real dog and resume her favourite hobby of rolling in cow dung.

I soon discovered I had badly underestimated how hard the work at the hospital would be.

A typical day as an equine intern starts at 6 am, though as the lowest in the hierarchy, by morning I had often already spent much of the night checking up on the 'hospital' patients in our care, changing bandages and providing medications every couple of hours. At 8 am there would be hospital rounds, not unlike what happens in a human hospital, during which I would follow around an equine specialist, a top-of-their-field professional, and report my assessment of each patient.

Patience was not a virtue of these senior vets, so to show any sign of weakness in your knowledge or hesitation in your reporting would be to incur their wrath. After surviving this daily mental pummelling, the next 8 to 12 hours was for the body to endure. The day was filled with administering anaesthetics for surgeries, assisting in lameness examinations, processing hospital admissions and conducting general consultations.

Days were long – 16 hours was common, 12 hours a 'light' day – plus the overnight work I mentioned and on-call weekends caring for hospital patients and dealing with emergency calls. It was an experience that would prepare me well for the sleep deprivation of motherhood, though I was looking after multiple 'babies' at once.

All this might have been easier to bear had the pay been okay. However, I was on a fixed salary that didn't account for all the overtime. At one point I worked out that, with the long hours, my earnings equated to around three dollars an hour.

Not all vet internships are like this. I have heard that small animal internships, especially those with a focus on exotic animals, are much kinder on mind and body. But horse care was for a long time perceived as being at the glamorous end of the veterinary profession, so there was never any shortage of keen young things ready to throw themselves to the lions, or whatever the equine equivalent is, and practices could afford to push us hard to sort the pretenders from the gladiators.

After six months of this I made what is still one of the most difficult decisions I've had to make in my career. I decided to leave the equine hospital. I was filled with disappointment in myself for not being able to cope with the job. It felt like failure. But vets are notoriously poor at putting their own health and wellbeing before their careers, and I decided that I was not willing to do that. The day I resigned I instantly felt the weight lift from my shoulders. I emerged, a shell of my former self, needing to find a way to rejuvenate and rebuild my confidence.

Now I was at a loose end. I was gun-shy about taking on another permanent position, and certainly wasn't ready to think about going out on my own. I needed a way to ease back into mixed-practice work without fear of finding myself locked into another position that would get on top of me. The obvious solution was to find some locum work and rebuild my confidence from there. I also needed to find somewhere to live.

While I worked out what to do, Mr Puss and I moved out of the unit and joined Kay and Brendan on his family's place near Kyabram. Brendan's bachelor pad was an old weatherboard house on the property. Picture the stereotypical bachelor's pad from the movies and this place would fit that image. Shower tiles with layers of soap scum, dishes washed on an as-needs basis, clothes stored on the 'floordrobe' rather than in a drawer, and certainly not hanging up. Having grown up with three sisters, he'd spent his childhood being waited on, hand and foot. Let's just say domestic cleanliness was not a high priority. But it was somewhere to stay when I had nowhere else.

There was one small issue we came up against with this move. The two farm dogs on the place had been trained to be hypervigilant about detecting pests like feral cats, rabbits and foxes. Mr Puss may have been a pedigree cat – he was a show-bred Ragdoll whose short legs had been considered disreputable to the breed, which is why he'd been offered for adoption – but these dogs didn't care about feline prestige. To them he was indistinguishable from a run-of-the-mill wild cat. After several confrontations, Mr Puss made clear that, while he may have been a pretty boy with his fluffy cream coat, white mittens and chocolate-pointed ears, he was not to be messed with. He came out unscathed, and a feline-canine truce was declared. The terms seemed to be that the dogs agreed not to eat Mr Puss as long as he remained inside the boundary of our yard.

Before long, Brendan's became a place to live on a more permanent basis. I managed to get a locum position with the

Kyabram Veterinary Clinic. The team at this practice were a vibrant, friendly and supportive group of people, just what I needed to help rebuild my confidence. It was another mixed practice, like Kerang, that included some clients with horses, so it was a comfortable environment in which to work. I was soon enjoying getting to know the locals and working with their animals. As I had in Kerang, I got involved in some local sport, including netball and touch football, which was a great way to make new friends.

As Brendan and I found ourselves cohabitating, my obsession with cleanliness started impose itself on his place. After a day scrubbing the shower, it was revealed that the bathroom tiles were, in fact, pure white. Brendan greeted this invasion of his previous life, from my pets to my cleaning habits, with the gentle, relaxed forbearance that I love about him. We settled into life under the same roof.

The stability of living with Brendan and settling into the vet clinic finally gave me the space to think about taking flying lessons. Getting started down this path would prove to be exactly what I needed to help get me out of my post-internship funk, not to mention move me closer to my ultimate goal. It helped that there was a good flying school just half an hour down the road at the Shepparton airport. This would become my second home for the next year or so.

Obtaining your pilot's licence in Australia has changed a lot over the years. I don't know what my grandfather had to do to get his licence, but I know my father was 19 or 20 when he got his. In those days, someone came to the property and conducted an introduction to flying on site, then Dad and his sister, along with a few others from the district, travelled down to Victoria to do their training.

These days, flight training, along with every aspect of aviation in Australia, is heavily regulated by the Civil Aviation Safety Authority. You obtain your licence in stages, the first being a Recreational Pilot Licence that allows you to fly on your own as long as you stay within 25 nautical miles of any airport you leave from. That obviously wasn't going to serve my dream of being a flying vet covering most of western New South Wales – it would barely get me out of our property! – so I needed to obtain my Private Pilot Licence. As well as learning how to actually fly a plane and logging the necessary hours in the air, I needed to undertake a substantial amount of study in the theory of flight, aerodynamics, aircraft knowledge, weather, navigation, flight planning, the laws of the air, and so on. All of this would ultimately be tested with a flying test and a written exam.

I chose to do the flying components of my training in a Cessna 172, the identical plane to my father's. While many people learn in lighter models of aircraft that can be more forgiving for beginners and are cheaper to operate (reducing the cost of lessons), my rationale was that I was never going to fly one of those planes in my practice so I might as well start on something closer to what I would be flying. And while it wasn't the plan that

I would use my father's plane as my practice aircraft, I couldn't look past the fact that there was already a Cessna taking up half the hanger at home and that there might be times when I'd need to borrow it if my plane was grounded for some reason.

Locum work allowed me to get off to a good start. The flexibility of being a casual employee meant that I could make the most of my flying time by having lessons early in the morning and when the weather was best. Trying to take advantage of this, I spent every spare moment at the aero club rooms. I could study there, talk to other students and instructors, and generally absorb as much information as possible. Aside from the time, the whole exercise was costing me all my income, so I was determined to make the most of every cent.

Meanwhile, at home, Brendan's acceptance of Kay and Mr Puss gave me an opening to introduce more pets. As a veterinarian, it is very difficult to abstain from animal hoarding. There are just so many critters that need a home. To date, other than Kay and Mr Puss, I had somehow restrained my predilection for collecting pets since leaving home, but now I was living somewhere with ample room, and with someone who was accepting, if not always enthusiastic, about having multiple animals around.

Mack and Gloria belonged to an elderly lady who had been breeding Burmese cats before she suffered a stroke and was placed in a nursing home. I was asked to euthanise her two remaining cats as there was nowhere for them to go. I recall walking into the backyard where the cattery stood – a large outdoor playpen structure that allowed the cats to play outside without straying from home.

As I entered the pen, I was met by a cream male cat who, despite his aged appearance, was bright-eyed and immediately brushed up against my legs like an old feline friend. My heart melted. I located his mate, a small, grey female, who was the opposite. She was timid, stand-offish and extremely overweight, though quick on her feet. She, too, won me over. I couldn't kill these animals. I *wouldn't* kill these animals. Instead, I sought the owner's permission, then bundled both cats into a carrier and took them back to the clinic for thorough health checks. Both had to be desexed and I wanted to ensure the female was not a diabetic. I also needed to check that they were free of any disease. By the time I returned to the clinic, the female cat had been named Gloria, which meant there was no turning back – they were mine from here on.

I took the two cats home that evening, arriving not long before Brendan.

'I might have done a thing,' I confessed, pointing to the cat carrier sitting on the coffee table.

'You've brought home a cat,' he said, finishing my confession for me.

He opened the door of the carrier to inspect them, and out came the male, followed by Gloria.

'No, I've brought home two cats,' I said with a grin, as Brendan shot me an incredulous look.

'This is Gloria,' I said, holding her up as if she were Simba in the opening scene of *The Lion King*. 'You can name the cream bloke.'

Thus Mack was named after a brand of truck.

Mack and Gloria enjoyed the best final years a retired breeding pair could wish for, spending their days sunning themselves on outdoor lounges then lazing on the couch with us for evening TV time.

I'd also long been keen to get another Australian terrier, the main breed of my childhood dog Bogan. Now, because I could, I got two. Walla and Bing, Aussie terrier puppies whose names were inspired by lyrics from the song 'Witch Doctor', came to us from separate breeders. They were each flown to Melbourne airport and I drove the three hours down there to pick them up. I still remember them as tiny little fuzz-balls, paddling down the corridor of the pet transporter's office towards me. At that age they could fit into the cup of my hands. Walla grew up to have a deep red in his wiry coat. He developed a habit of running into things at full pace, simply because he didn't look where he was going. Bing, with his blue coat, smokey black body, and tan paws and face, became, at once, both extremely cute and a serial killer of mice, chooks, pigeons and, more recently, snakes.

The constant through all this was Kay. The two of us spent a good 12 years together before she developed an incurable spinal tumour. It was a small consolation that her condition deteriorated rapidly, so she didn't have a prolonged period of suffering.

Later, Walla experienced a common misfortune of little dogs in the bush, coming off second best after an altercation with a king brown snake. We found him lying under the house with the body of the snake nearby. He had passed before we realised what had happened. I always have a stash of anti-venom on hand, but it's of no use when the victim is already deceased.

Brendan was deeply upset at the loss of Walla, who had been his first pet dog. We buried Walla in the sandhill beside our house, his collar twitched to the top of a fencepost marking his grave. We've often thought about ways of preventing snakes and dogs crossing paths, but in the end we have to accept that what will be will be. You cannot stop a dog from living its life. Better they live a good, short life than a long, caged one.

There was one other cat that very nearly joined the team at Brendan's house, but was saved from that outcome (or, rather, Brendan was) by one of our surgery nurses taking it on. It had quite a journey before it got to that point though.

I try not to intervene in the final decisions of an owner. However, on the day a client brought in a kitten that we had recently diagnosed with a portosystemic shunt, I had to refuse their request to euthanise the animal. The condition is one in which the animal is born with a blood vessel open that should have closed at birth, resulting in blood that is supposed to flow to the liver bypassing ('shunting') around it instead. Ultimately this results in liver failure unless the problem is corrected. That involves some pretty groovy surgery, during which a cellophane tube is fitted around the persistent duct (the erroneously open blood vessel) using a minute camera with remote controls. The cellophane progressively shrinks, slowly closing off the shunt.

In this case, the owners could not afford such specialist care – a perfectly understandable situation as the surgery required is expensive. However, when I stared down at the euthanasia permission form, I couldn't bring myself to do it. Instead, I suggested that the owner surrender the kitten into my care, releasing all ownership, and I would see what I could do. The man and his son were grateful that I had offered them another option, and I was relieved they were willing to take it, though in truth I knew I couldn't afford the treatment either. Nevertheless, I was determined to do my good deed for the feline species.

I contacted an animal rescue group, who took pity upon my new little friend and offered to take her in and pay for her lifesaving surgery.

'We've got an appointment organised with the specialists in Melbourne next week,' the lady in charge of the organisation told me over the phone. 'Would you mind looking after her until then?'

I readily agreed, offering to take the kitten into the city to deliver her to the specialist clinic. Over the next few days we looked after the cat, while being careful not to give her a name.

When the day came for her to travel down to Melbourne, Brendan and I planned to make the trip by rail. It wasn't until we got to the station that I realised animals were not on allowed on the train. This required some quick thinking. I took the cat out of its carrier and threw it back into the car. That would be a dead giveaway. I then emptied my large handbag and placed a blanket inside it, placed the little kitty on the blanket and closed the bag enough that the cat couldn't stick her head out. Satisfied, we boarded the train, trying to look completely normal.

Sitting in the carriage, I prayed our friend wouldn't make a single meow. Thankfully, her silence lasted until well after the conductor had been through our car, though after that she started to make some squeaky protests. I pulled her out and sat her on my lap, hoping no one would dob us in. I was surprised when we didn't get a single comment from any onlookers – no one seemed the least bit nonplussed by the presence of a cat in the carriage. One lady sitting opposite eventually commented on how adorable the little kitten was. That was it.

After we pulled into Southern Cross Station, I realised that this was where the challenge was really going to be. Without the carrier, we now had to carry a cat in a handbag through the middle of Melbourne's central business district. Fortune smiled on my bold manoeuvre. We made it through the bustling station and out onto the footpath, where we flagged down a taxi, hurriedly climbing in before our own passenger could escape. I decided not to tell the taxi driver about his stowaway, as I was pretty sure pets aren't allowed in taxis either. Eventually, though, the inevitable noises of annoyance started coming from my bag.

'My phone makes the strangest noises since I changed my settings,' I said in response to a bemused look from the driver.

The taxi finally pulled up in front of the specialist clinic, where I left Brendan to pay the fare as I rushed inside the building. I approached the young receptionist, who gave me a quizzical look when, to him, it looked as though I'd arrived for my appointment without the actual patient.

'She's in my handbag,' I said sheepishly, cracking opening the top of the bag to show him.

He called for a nurse, who took the cat in her arms and carried her straight through to the ward cages.

'Who is the referring vet?' asked the receptionist as he took down the details.

'That would be me,' I replied.

He gave me that look – the 'you are completely bat-shit crazy' look.

Though I suppose I'd asked for that. The real truth is that, if it weren't for Brendan, I would really be crazy, and likely the owner of 20 cats who had been rejected for one reason or other. If crazy meant giving a cat a train ride in a handbag, I could live with that.

The good news is that our efforts were rewarded. The kitten made a full recovery after the specialist surgery, and eventually started its new life with my colleague.

*

Flying lessons included a lot of time spent going over checklists and procedures, and a lot of practice of the main steps in any flight, regardless of its length: take off, cruise and landing.

Taxiing and taking off are relatively straightforward, as are cruising and manoeuvring in the air – at least in smooth air. The more challenging part is landing, because that involves good judgment and finesse of the controls, especially the flaps, as you nurse the plane onto the runway. Extending the flaps slows the aircraft while providing a steep but controllable descent; knowing when and how much to deploy them is an important part of the pilot's 'touch'. The aim when landing is to bring the engine to an idle just above the surface, pull the nose up, then glide the plane down so that its rear wheels gently kiss the tarmac just past the runway's threshold. When you get that right, it's bliss. Every pilot, even commercial jet pilots, will give themselves an internal pat on the back when they nail it. When you get it wrong, the wheels thumping hard into the surface or, worse, bouncing off it, well, those are the times you hope no one is watching.

There were a couple of sheds not far back from the start of the airstrip where I learnt to fly. From mid-morning on a warm day, the heat would radiate off the tin roofs of those sheds, pushing the air upwards. So often I would have a landing perfectly set up, the plane's position and controls just right, when I'd get a bump from that rising air, sending my plans out of kilter. That was all part of the learning, of course, as was dealing with other conditions like the direction and strength of the wind. You do a *lot* of circuits during your training, with the specific purpose of practising landings.

The other thing we practised a lot during our lessons were emergency drills. After covering the basics, instructors take great pleasure in randomly pulling the throttle back to idle and saying, 'Righto, you've lost your engine. Where are you going to land?' Eventually you get to the point that you choose your spot, then actually go to make the landing, getting quite close to the ground before powering up and heading back into the sky. Learning in the country meant there were usually plenty of paddocks to choose from as potential emergency landing strips, but being in a relatively populated area of countryside meant there were also powerlines everywhere.

You really don't want to hit a powerline, both because of the 'tripping hazard' they present to the wheels and also, of course, the risk of electrocution. Often these aren't obvious from the air, so what looks like a nice open paddock suddenly becomes a death trap as you get closer and realise there is a single strand of power cable stretching right across its middle. Before long you get better practiced at identifying these earlier.

You practise emergency procedures so much that, by the time you get your licence, you're convinced that aeroplanes drop out of the sky virtually every second. The reality is that engine failure is extremely rare, but there aren't any second chances when you're in the sky. Should you find yourself in an actual emergency, these routines need to be second nature so that you can follow them without panicking.

The hardest part of my tuition wasn't actually flying, but learning all the mechanical and aeronautical stuff, which really isn't my gig. Physics was something I thought I'd left behind me at school, and learning the parts of an engine was completely new to me. Fortunately, I had Brendan, qualified fitter and turner and keen mechanic, on hand to patiently guide me through that stuff.

Every learner pilot's initial goal – indeed their dream – is their first solo flight. Think of the first time you drove a car on your own, without an instructor or parent beside you, and multiply that feeling by a hundred. Virtually all aeroplanes other than the smallest have 'dual controls', meaning the yoke or stick and pedals used to control the plane in the air are duplicated on the co-pilot side. That means that if you mess up as a student pilot, your instructor can take over in an instant. While they rarely do that as you become more experienced, the backup is always there … until that first solo flight. Once you get up in the air on your own, you are really on your own. Screw up and you'll face the consequences. There's nowhere to hide, and all that. As if to emphasis your solitude, the plane even behaves slightly differently because it is carrying 80kg less, give or take, which is significant in a light aircraft.

Where Dad and his sister had been allowed to do their first solo flight after logging 12 hours with an instructor, I needed to log a minimum of 20 hours before taking my first solo flight. My instructor also needed to be satisfied that I was ready. Dad being Dad, that meant I was badgered constantly as I approached the 20-hour mark, him wanting to know when the solo would come and reminding me how quickly he'd done his.

When it did come, it was without fanfare. One morning, I was out doing circuits with my instructor, Nathan. A circuit is a basic training run. You take off, reach your intended altitude, then draw a rectangle in the sky before lining up the runway to land at the opposite end from where you took off. After touching down, instead of pulling off the runway, you power up, take off again and repeat the whole process. I'd flown two or three circuits before, while we were still rolling after landing, Nathan said, 'Alright, I'll stop you here.' He opened his door and stepped out, then said, 'Okay, off you go. Do a couple of laps on your own.'

I digested what he said, turned the plane around and taxied back to the top of the runway to take off. I was nervous but also confident, as you want to be. I'd done dozens of laps by now, so I did know what I was doing. I talked myself through all the take off steps then, as I reached altitude, I settled into the feeling of being on my own in the sky. There really is nothing like the feeling of ultimate freedom this gives you. I started singing to myself and soaking it all up. It was a great feeling, and even though I spend so much time in the sky on my own these days, I'll never forget that first time.

Unfortunately, successfully completing your first solo doesn't make you a licensed pilot. I still had plenty of hours of flying to go, with an increasing focus on navigation skills. And I still had the theoretical side to finish. It would take me 12 months to earn my Private Pilot Licence. On the day of my final examination, I was more nervous than I had been for my final veterinary science exams. The chief flying instructor, Alan Cole, took advantage of my nervous state as he listed the airfields that he wanted me to navigate my way around. There was one I hadn't heard of, so I asked him, 'How do you spell that?'

'T. H. A. T,' he said.

I had written the word on my list before I realised I'd fallen for the oldest dad joke in the book!

Thankfully I passed the test and was awarded my 'wings'. I was officially a pilot as well as a vet. Now to find a way to bring the two together.

HITCHED

Towards the end of 2016, Brendan and I had been dating for two years and living together for one, and I was impatiently awaiting a proposal of marriage. I had thought the question might be popped on the weekend after I'd received my wings, but no such luck. After that I took to openly googling diamond rings and even leaving the occasional picture on the fridge door, but still there was nothing.

One weekend we went horse riding and camping in the Victorian High Country with some local friends, Brett and Clare. We rode to Craig's Hut, the shack perched high on Mount Buller that was built as a set for, and made famous by, the movie *The Man from Snowy River*. Brett and Clare had been married at this beautiful place and they were now celebrating an anniversary back up there. But if I thought any of the romance of this was going to rub off on Brendan, I was to be disappointed. As we began our ride back down the mountain, it sank in that no grand gesture would be forthcoming.

Perhaps Brendan might eventually propose in, oh, 50 years, with a ring made of fencing wire twitched into a circle. In the meantime I'd just have to wait.

So I was bewildered when the proposal did finally come.

I was in Echuca playing touch football. It was a hot day in February, and I'd just come off the field after my game. My clothes were grubby, I was sweaty and stinky, I had sunscreen smothered into all my exposed skin, and my hair was pulled up into a greasy bun atop my head. In short, sexy and romantic I was not.

Brendan had come up in his own car to watch the game and greeted me with an ice cream, which was very welcome. We sat on the bank of the Murray River, licking our treats while I cooled down. At one point, Brendan took my hand, looked at me and popped the question.

I paused; it was a bit of a deer-in-the-headlights moment. I had been waiting for this, as I've said, but I was not expecting it to happen on this day, and certainly not over ice creams in my football gear.

'Can I think about it?' I answered. Yes, I was that person. After badgering him for months about wanting a ring, I now wanted a minute to collect myself. At the least I wanted to not be the greasy, stinky mess I was in that moment. I wasn't going to become engaged smelling like dirty socks! I wanted to have a shower and get into some clean clothes.

Unfortunately, having come in separate cars, we each had to drive home on our own, in our own thoughts. Brendan went ahead of me while I cleaned myself up, and by the time I got home he was in sulk mode. He really didn't get where I was coming from.

I came up with a plan for how to respond to his proposal.

I wrote a note on a small piece of paper and rolled it up, tucking it into Mack's collar just before we sat down for TV time. It was a nice touch, I thought, choosing the cat that Brendan had named to be my messenger. Mack and Gloria took up their customary spot in the middle of the couch, Brendan and I taking up our positions either side, Brendan next to Mack. He began stroking the cat but, after several minutes, he still hadn't found the note.

'What's that under Mack's collar?' I asked, trying to be nonchalant.

Brendan, still with the shits, just shrugged. I urged him again. With a sigh, he scratched around the cat's collar and pulled out the note:

In answer to your question, YES!

VARYING VALUES

One night a few months later, I was woken from my slumber by the blaring ringtone of the after-hours phone. I fumbled in the darkness to find it. As I answered the call, I managed to peel my eyes open and look at the time: 1.30 am!

The dairy farmer on the line, Mr Smith, had a heifer cow that was having difficulty calving. On the upside, he was only ten minutes away. On the downside, it was the middle of winter in northern Victoria, which meant wet and bitterly cold. *Why did I give up living in the desert for this?* I grumbled to myself as I clambered out of my warm bed, glancing enviously over towards Brendan, who was asleep in his cocoon, blissfully unaware that I was even awake.

I heaved on some thick overalls and a rainproof vest, then stepped out of the house into a thrashing wind and a sleety drizzle. Mr Puss was curled up with Bing and Walla on the dog bed outside the kitchen door, feline and canines putting their differences aside to survive the brutal chill. None of them even raised an ear as I started the car, turned the heater on full-bore, and reversed out of the garage. As I drove towards the Smiths' farm, I thought that I would like to be a vet's pet in my next life, lazing about all day with a doctor at my beck and call.

I turned down the dirt road into the Smiths' farm, now made muddy from the rain. The car slipped a little, but I managed to stay on the road, and soon a floodlight at the dairy shed revealed Mr Smith's short frame and mop of curly hair against the darkness of the night.

As I wound down my window to greet him, the rain whipped me in the face. I squinted as I shook hands through the open window.

'She's down in the calving paddock behind the dairy,' he said. He was dressed in a raincoat and gumboots. He walked ahead of me with a torch as I followed in the car, driving down the lane beside the shed. After Mr Smith opened the gate and I drove through, I could make out the heifer sitting down in the middle of the small, muddy paddock. I pulled up with the nose of the car pointing at the young cow, the headlights illuminating the scene.

Mr Smith arrived at my side as I gathered all the equipment I needed from the back of the car. He had already placed a bucket of warm, clean water beside the back end of the heifer. We trudged through the mud to her tail end and I knelt down in the squelch as I pulled my gloves on. After I administered an epidural and muscle relaxant, the farmer poured some lubricant over my arms and I inserted them inside the cow's vagina. Her pelvic cavity was a surreal warm reprieve from the bitter cold as I felt my way around and built up an image of what was going on. It wasn't good.

The heifer had rammed the calf tight up against the pelvis so that all I could feel was one slimy shoulder of the foetus. While the calf was coming forward, as it should have been, there was only one foot in the birthing canal. Its head and the other front leg were tucked under the body and would have to be released for any hope of a successful birth.

Under normal circumstances I would have let out a stream of profanity at this point. If there's one thing I was gifted by the males I grew up around, it was a talent for swearing like a sailor when things are going pear-shaped. However, I knew from past experience that this sort of language would not be appreciated by Mr Smith. He was a very active member of the local community church and did not abide cursing or the use of the Lord's name in vain.

For now, I kept my swearing to myself.

This was going to be a difficult calving. I explained to Mr Smith that the calf was unlikely to be alive as it had probably suffocated due to the awkward position of its head. Nevertheless, it still had to come out. I tried for what felt like hours to reposition it, but despite my best efforts and all the medications I could use to relax the uterus, it became clear that there was no way I was going to able to manipulate the calf into a more natural birthing position. After a while I couldn't keep my language inside anymore, however I managed to stick to words like 'lovey', 'darling' and 'fudgecake'. These words had none of the cathartic effect of my usual repertoire.

Finally, it was time to consider other options for removing the foetus. The drizzle was getting heavier and the paddock muddier, so performing a caesarean section and withdrawing the calf through the flank was not an option. The rain and mud would contaminate the sterility of the surgery, most certainly leading to an abdominal infection and a painful death for the cow.

This left only one option. It was clear by now that the calf was already dead, but I could save the cow by performing a fetotomy. This is a somewhat gruesome procedure involving dissection of the foetus inside the pelvis using a serrated fetotomy wire, removing the calf a piece at a time. While it sounds very unpleasant, procedures like this are a reality of being a large-animal vet. Why lose both cow and calf when one could be saved? (Nevertheless, feel free to skip down to the next break if you need to.)

I discussed what I had to do with Mr Smith. By now the cold was beginning to seep through my wet overalls, but I needed to lie in the mud on my belly in order to reach my hand in deep enough to pass the fetotomy wire around the neck of the foetus. My right arm was in up to my shoulder, my head leaning up against the cow's vulva. I was practically swimming in the mud as I managed to successfully place the cutting wire. With a burst of energy, I leaned back, vigorously pulling the wire back and forth. Suddenly I fell onto my buttocks as the cut was complete.

After reaching in to check that the head was indeed separate from the body, I attached the calving ropes to the leg that remained extended in the pelvic canal. Mr Smith and I both put all our weight into tugging on the leg, but it didn't budge.

'Bloody hell!' I cried in frustration.

'No need to use such language,' said Mr Smith.

I turned to him, almost out of patience and energy. He wasn't the one tired, freezing and covered in mud.

'That is the most polite curse word I've got,' I said. 'I have much worse words I could use. I think a few "bloodys" and "buggers" are allowed in these circumstances.'

'You don't go to church, do you?' said Mr Smith. 'You should join us sometime.'

I wasn't sure how to respond to that without offending the man, so I said nothing, kneeling in the mud and easing myself back onto my belly to have another feel inside the vagina. It was tight and my hand was going numb with the pressure on it as I attempted to reach underneath, between the foetus and the wall of the uterus. And was it possible to be any colder?

There are days in every vet's career where you seriously consider taking on a different profession. This was one of those days for me, and it wasn't even dawn.

'I'll have to perform a subcutaneous fetotomy.'

I explained the procedure by which I would remove the skin of the front leg, which would then allow easy removal of the leg itself. I got underway with the messy task and was able to pull the leg off with another tug on the calving rope. Kneeling once more to feel within the uterus, I located the other leg wedged underneath the pelvic brim, the inside edge of the pelvic bone. By now my strength was waning, so when I attempted to grasp the slimy leg and pull it forward, I was too weak to hold on. I tried over and over, muttering more than a few bloodys and buggers as I went.

'How much longer will this take? I have to start milking at four,' said Mr Smith.

I looked up as I lost my grip on the leg once more.

I was beaten.

'I don't have the strength left in me to get the leg up and out,' I said. 'We'll call it a night and I'll return in the morning to get the rest of the foetus out.'

'Let's pray over her a while,' came the farmer's suggestion.

'You do that,' I said, the last of my patience gone. 'I'm going to go home for a shower and some rest. I'll be back at 8 am to finish the job so the cow can survive.'

It was 4.30 am when I got to the shower. I crawled back into my bed after setting several alarms to ensure I woke up. I don't think I'd ever been so exhausted.

Barely had my head hit the pillow, or so it felt, then the alarm jolted me awake. Still, the rest had restored enough energy to get me back to the farm.

With one Herculean effort, the foetus popped out from the vagina. I propped the heifer up onto her sternum, offering her a warm drink of electrolytes from a bucket, which she gratefully drank in deep gulps.

Job done.

Unfortunately, the vet industry is one in which there's no such thing as having a day off after pulling an all-nighter at work. I had a full diary of farm calls ahead of me. I would get through it fuelled by caffeine and fast food, my self-prescribed treat after the nightmarish night before. Coffee is my addiction, the least harmful of all the bad habits I could take up, I figure.

The local cafes in Kyabram knew me and the other vets well, especially during calving season when we would drop in frequently for takeaway. Often the barista would sit a little treat atop the plastic lid, passing over the coffee with a kind smile as if to say, 'Hang in there, mate, you can do this.' Aside from coffee, a power nap for a couple of minutes here and there – and perhaps 30 minutes lying in the dark of the X-ray room over lunch – would help keep me functioning until the end of my shift.

Having just completed what I thought was my last job for the day, I was walking into the office at the vet clinic to sit down and write up my patient notes. I flicked on the kettle in the smoko room, readying myself for an hour of typing on the computer. Just as I did so, the receptionist put her head around the door with a look of sympathy.

'I'm afraid I have a call out for you,' she said. 'Mr Smith has requested you specifically. He has another calving.'

My heart sank as the kettle boiled teasingly beside me. I shrugged, a feeling of foreboding settling on my shoulders.

'Tell him I'll be there in 15,' I said.

I dragged myself out the back door of the clinic and pulled on my gumboots while striving to bolster my enthusiasm. At least it was still daylight.

The cow that Mr Smith had waiting for me was upright on all fours. That was a welcome sight at the end of a long day. I wasn't going swimming in the mud this time. I noted that Mr Smith was in a jovial mood as we guided the cow into the crush behind the dairy shed.

I donned my usual calving garb, my shoulder-length gloves and rubber apron, and felt around inside the birth canal. The calf was coming backwards, however both hindlegs were in the correct position in the canal for a breech birth. I was relieved, though on feeling more thoroughly, I realised it would take some effort to assist with this delivery as it was a large calf.

I conveyed this to Mr Smith, who nodded in reply. I busied myself setting up a calving pulley and attaching the ropes that would hopefully make the job easier.

'Why aren't you a believer?' said Mr Smith.

'I'm just not the religious type,' I replied, concentrating on the job at hand.

Undeterred, he began to explain the ways of the Lord. I tried to ignore him, but the man became more enthusiastic as he delivered a crush-side sermon, with me as a literal captive audience. His behaviour was so different from that of the soft-spoken man I knew him as.

'I'm not completely atheist,' I said, trying to politely avoid his pronouncements without adding fuel to his fire. 'My fiancé's family are religious and go to church every week.'

Would that be enough to excuse me?

'What religion are they?' he asked.

'Catholic,' I said as I started tugging on the calving pulley. As I thought, the calf was going to take a bit of time to extract.

'They don't count,' he retorted.

Great, I thought. I handed him the rope for the calving pulley.

'If you could put your *ethereal* energies into helping deliver this calf, that would be most helpful,' I said.

He got the hint, although his sermon continued even as, after what felt like an eternity, the calf plopped out. I broke its fall to ensure a gentle arrival to the world. The little calf bellowed as I cleared its airways of birthing mucous, then we let the cow out of the crush and into the yard so that she could clean her newborn.

Day done. At last.

I packed up my equipment and made ready to leave, but after he asked once again why I wasn't a believer, I snapped.

'Look,' I began, annoyed that after all this time he hadn't perceived my disinterest. 'You might like going to church on a Saturday night and praying. I like going to the pub, getting a gutful of grog and going home to have premarital sex. And that isn't going to change.'

Sudden and total silence descended.

I placed my equipment into the vet car and got in behind the wheel.

'Good evening,' I said through the car window. Mr Smith said not a word. As I drove off he stood still, dumbfounded and mouth agape.

I attended to Mr Smith's farm many times after that occasion. I didn't feel great about how I'd left him that day, but on the plus side he never bothered to give me a religious sermon again.

BIG RED

In mid-2017, I was offered an ongoing position as an associate vet with the Kyabram clinic. I'd already done numerous locum stints with them over the previous two years, interspersed with other locums, including a few months in south-east Queensland. Now, with my confidence restored and well-established roots in the area, I was ready for permanent work again. I took the role on with enthusiasm and continued to work with the local characters, building up my skills – and collecting the occasional injury – as a settled rural vet.

I can't reveal the name of the town where this first story takes place, because to do so might be to put the main character into jeopardy. Suffice to say that it's a sleepy town on the bank of a muddy river. Old sandstone buildings hint at the town's former glory, times when it bustled with activity. These days it's just another place on the road where you're forced to slow down. A major state highway cuts though the centre of town, so trucks rumble through at all hours. The occasional tourist pauses to get fuel and take a photo of the river as they pass over the bridge.

There seem to be more pets than people. You rarely see a human walking on the pavement, but semi-domesticated pets roam the streets day and night. The villagers are accustomed to pets roaming free, so long as little harm is done, though the council ranger is kept busy collecting the strays. Most of the free-roaming animals are dogs and cats, though the occasional hen braves the sidewalk, pecking at fresh grass clippings after the council has mowed the nature strips. These free-range hens don't tend to wander far from their coops, the threat of four-legged company keeping them within a defined territory.

One bird was a very obvious exception. A large Rhode Island Red rooster with dark green tail feathers, an orange breast and bold red comb, he was hard to miss. He made for a glorious sight strutting proudly along fence lines, casting a stern eye over inferior animals about town.

While the talk around most country towns is filled with gossip and differences of opinion, Big Red, as he became known, gave this township something they could all agree on. He was a pest. *Gallus non grata*. The reason wasn't his arrogance, but his ill-timed crowing.

It didn't matter whether it was 2 am or 2 pm. Big Red voiced his presence whenever he felt the urge – loud and proud, morning, noon and night. What he hoped to achieve by this I couldn't say, but he was always ranging about solo, so presumably he wasn't impressing any of the local hens.

No one claimed ownership of this bird, and all attempts to catch him had failed. Each time I visited the town there was a new story about Big Red's latest close encounter with entrapment.

At one stage, the local ranger was so bombarded by requests that the job became his top priority for a whole week. He drove about town daily, from the start to the end of his shift, searching for Big Red.

On the first day of his mission, he found the bird in the town's local park during the mid-afternoon, the bird seeking refuge from the afternoon heat amongst the gumtrees that dotted the riverside reserve. The ranger laid a trap using chook pellets for bait, but at the end of the day all he had were a few innocently imprisoned, and rightly grumpy, cockatoos.

The ranger then decided on another tactic. He would befriend the bird, in order to get close enough to place a net or dog-catching pole around him. He started having his afternoon smoko in the park. After a few afternoons, Big Red became accustomed to sharing the shade with the ranger, and even accepted a few crumbs of cake. Slowly, the ranger introduced the dog-catching pole into the scene, laying it on the ground with the noose open. The plan was that eventually the bird would wander over the noose, and at that moment the ranger would pull the loop tight, firmly encircling Big Red's foot.

This plan worked. After much commotion and ruffling of feathers, the ranger managed to wrestle the rooster into the back of his van. He patted himself on the back as he returned to the pound, taking his time on the drive down the main street as a sort of victory parade.

As he neared the council offices, he noted that Big Red's crowing, which had been muffled by the canopy on the back of his wagon, seemed to have become a bit clearer. A bit further on, a group of Aboriginal kids playing on the footpath started laughing and pointing.

'Mister, the bird is on your roof,' they said.

The ranger stopped the vehicle to see what was going on. Big Red had managed to squeeze out through the air vent of the vehicle's canopy and was perched upon the opening, enjoying a free ride down the street. To add insult to injury, the rooster proceeded to empty his bowels onto the top of the car, before flapping his wings and flying over a high fence into a private back yard.

The story of Big Red's capture and escape quickly spread through town. The community soon resolved to deal with the problem themselves.

Traps of varied and sometimes novel design started popping up in backyards all over town. Some tried to use cat traps, but Big Red was too clever to be caught in one of those. A class at the local school invented their own trap, tethering a milk crate in a tree above an offering of bird treats, with plans to release the rope holding the trap when Big Red took the bait. It took several weeks, but eventually, after replacing the offerings multiple times, they discovered his favourite snack was deep fried chips from the school tuckshop.

One lunchtime they spied Big Red having a munch and set the crate loose. It fell neatly over the top of the rooster, but the children's joy didn't last long. The bird simply stood up straight, shook the crate off and ran for it. Several children tried to leap on him, but he evaded their tackles like a seasoned rugby player and made his escape. He was not seen near the school yard again.

The longer the chase for Big Red went on, the more kudos was on offer for any local who could catch him. Could anyone achieve what was increasing looking like an impossibility?

I'd heard a lot about Big Red's exploits from Valerie, who ran the local post office, which was a convenient place to leave medications for clients who couldn't meet me face to face. Valerie was a cheerful woman in her mid-sixties, with a gleaming blonde bob and bright lipstick. She had moved to town ten years previously, in search of a quieter and less costly life. After buying a house, her plan had been to see out her days in semi-retirement. That idea proved short-lived after she took on the full-time job of managing the post office. Still, compared to working in a city, she found this job a lot less demanding and the slower pace much less tiring.

It proved to be a great way for Valerie to become involved in the community, and the perfect way to stay abreast of local news and gossip. There wasn't much Valerie didn't know. She wasn't prone to gossiping herself, but if you asked her if she'd heard anything on some topic, she would readily volunteer any information she had.

I enjoyed the brief chats I had with Valerie. It was rare to go into the post office and find no one else there, even if they were just sitting in the corner reading a newspaper. Valerie was very patient with those who tended to outstay their welcome, clearly enjoying the company.

One day I was chatting to Valerie while a couple of other people browsed the post office store's offerings. I sensed that there was something she wanted to talk to me about, but that the presence of others in the room was preventing her from speaking up. As I left, I handed her my business card.

'Give me a buzz, or feel free to share my details with anyone who needs veterinary assistance,' I said.

Within five minutes, Valerie rang me.

'Thank you,' she said. 'I had no idea how to ask you this in case someone overheard.'

Then she dropped a bombshell.

'I'm the one who's been looking after that rooster everyone's hell-bent on capturing.'

I took a deep breath. So there was someone the rooster trusted? That was a surprise.

'Right Val,' I said. 'Never fear. Your secret is safe with me.'

'I figured as much. I've noticed that you're always confidential in the way you conduct yourself.'

'Part of the job,' I said. 'What can I help you with?'

Valerie told me that she thought Big Red may have broken a foot during his most recent escape. He was limping about. We arranged to meet that evening after the post office had closed. It happened to be grand final night, so most people had their attention well away from the post office. As I drove over, I reflected on what a tremendous actress Valerie must be, staying nonchalant whenever someone spoke of Big Red's latest escape.

In the backyard of the post office, in the fading light, I found Valerie sitting on a garden bench with Big Red sitting beside her. I greeted them both with an amused smile.

'Who'd have thought a street bird could be so docile,' I said.

'Yes – like a child on best behaviour for their mum.'

I got Valerie to cuddle the bird as I checked him over. Apart from the issue with his leg, he appeared to be in excellent health. His gleaming feathers, even in this low light, were a good sign.

'I think it's his left leg that he's been limping on,' Valerie said.

Right on cue, Big Red let out a shriek of protest as I felt that leg, or more specifically his foot. The foot also looked slightly swollen.

'Well, it's hard to tell if he's broken a bone in there,' I said, 'and my X-ray is too powerful for this little leg. It would probably radiate it to smithereens. But it's clearly quite painful. I reckon I'll pop a really good bandage on it, with a little cast around it to provide stability until it sets.'

When I gave the rooster a pain relief injection, he took it stoically. I wrapped the foot with a small bandage and plenty of padding so that he wouldn't get any rub marks. I then placed a small amount of plastic casting bandage around his foot. Ideally, I would get the owner to confine an animal with a bandaged leg, but in this case it clearly wasn't going to happen. The material was light enough that it wouldn't affect Big Red's ability to fly away.

Once I was done, Valerie popped him onto the ground, where he strutted around with a slight limp.

'He already looks better!' Val proclaimed.

'Give it a couple of weeks and then remove that bandage. In the meantime, if you notice him looking sore or limping more, take the bandage off. A bandage that rubs won't do him any good.'

I gave her a bottle of liquid pain relief and asked her to administer it daily for the next few weeks. Then I crossed my fingers that the bandage wouldn't slip.

I emerged from the backyard and looked down the street. No one in sight. You could have fired a shotgun without a soul hearing. I was satisfied my mission had remained a secret.

As it happened, I was back in this town only about a week later. As I refuelled my car, the ranger pulled up beside me. He hefted out of his seat and wandered around towards me, leaning on the passenger side as I filled up.

I looked up casually.

'G'day Kev, what's going on?'

'I reckon someone owns Big Red,' he said, leaning over towards me.

'Is that so?' I replied, keeping a cool tone and not bothering to look up from my task.

'I reckon he must have seen a vet,' Kev continued.

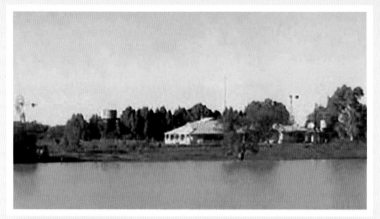

The homestead on our property, as seen across the lake.

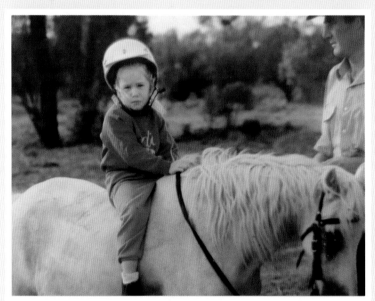

An early horse ride with Dad holding my horse.

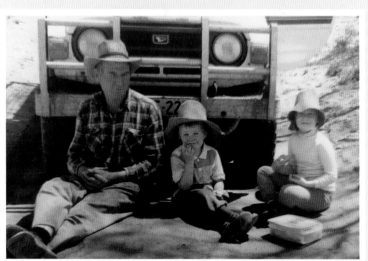

Dad, James, and me having a snack in the red dirt of the homestead. James is wearing one of Dad's retired Akubras.

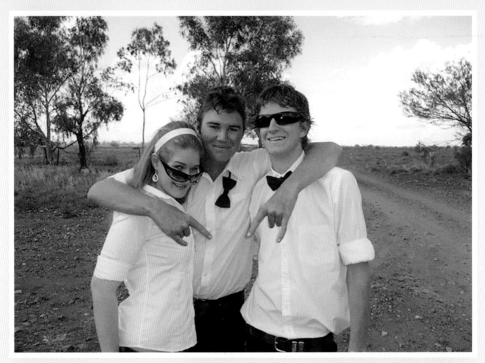

Me, James, and his friend, Mitchell. Both boys were killed together in a car accident.

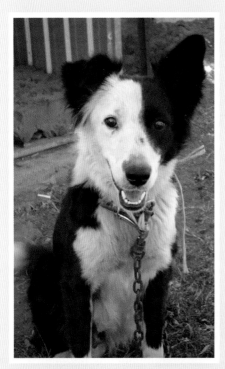

Kay, who got me through a lot in my youth.

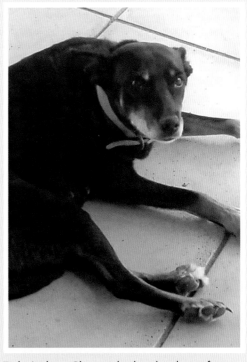

Ticka's dog, Chips, who lived with us after Ticka passed away.

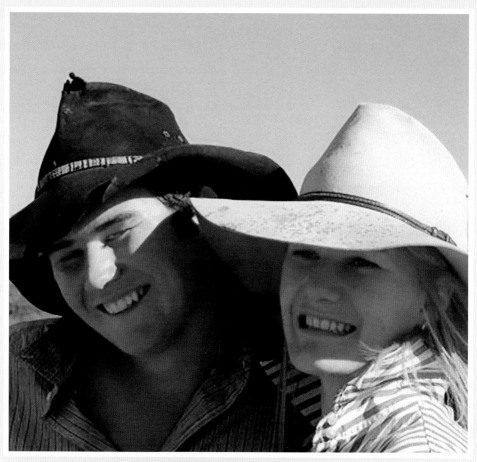

James and me, out of and in the water.

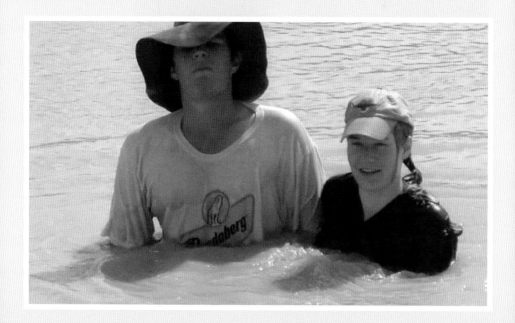

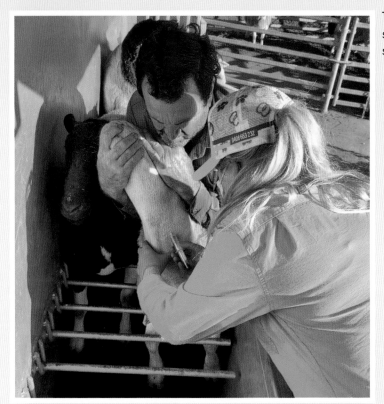

Taking a blood sample from a sheep.

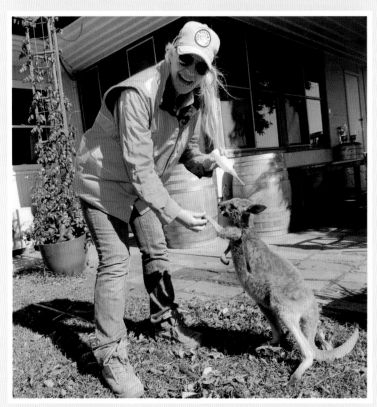

Making friends with a rescued roo.

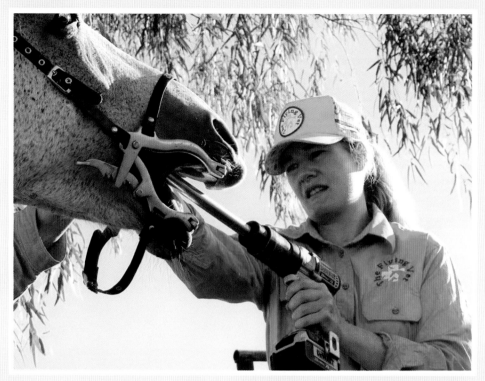

Tooth-grinding with the drill. Dentistry at large scale!

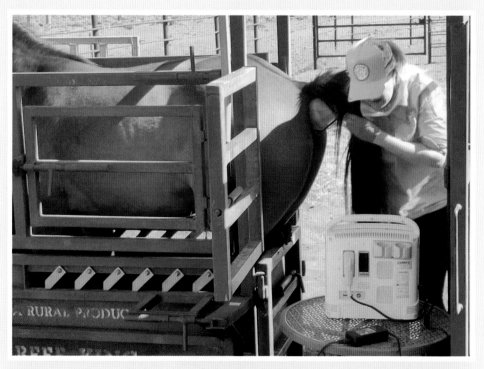

Pregnancy testing. I've been in this position thousands of times with cattle and horses.

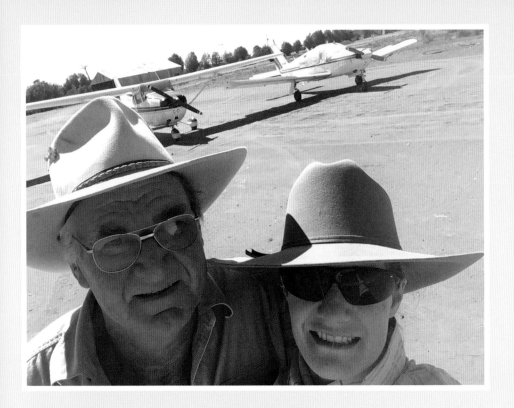

Dad and me in front of our planes.

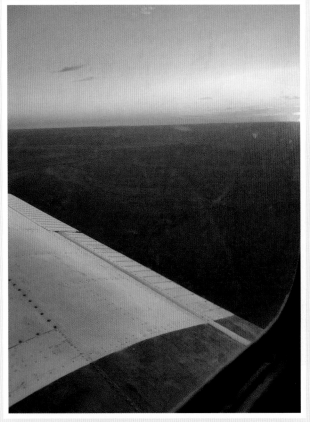

There's nothing like the sight of a sunrise seen from your own aeroplane.

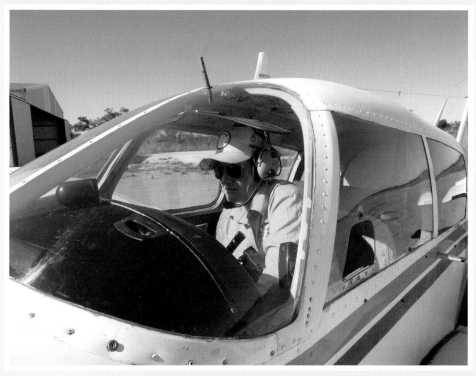

In the cockpit of my lovely Piper Arrow.

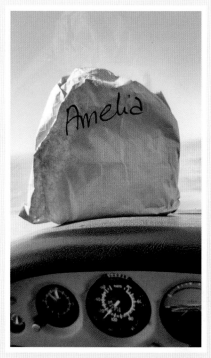

Lunch for the road. Well ... the air!

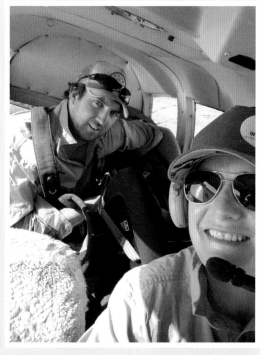

Family outing in the Piper, with me at the controls, Brendan and baby Lindsay in the back.

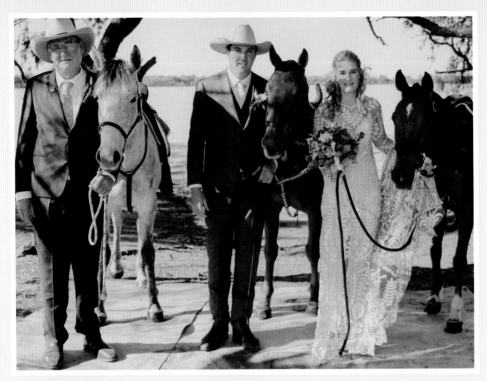

Our wedding day – a country affair. *(Courtesy Jayde Creative Photography)*

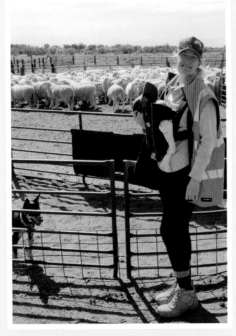

Lindsay's early introduction to farming.

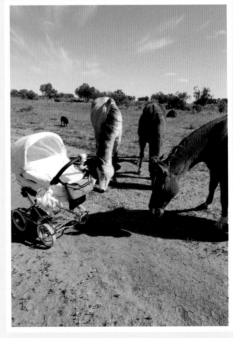

Equine babysitters.

'Really, what makes you think that?' I said, feigning surprise as I looked up.

'He's got a bandage on his leg.'

I paused.

'From what I hear he's a pretty smart chook. Perhaps he wrapped himself up.'

I gave the ranger a cheeky wink, replaced the fuel cap and hung the nozzle on the bowser before excusing myself. I had a busy day ahead of me.

ALL I WANT FOR CHRISTMAS

The noise the gate made as it clanged into my mouth was similar to that of a porcelain cup breaking. My beautiful pearly whites were shattered. Years of dental care and thousands of dollars spent on braces to get them into a neat formation, ruined in an instant.

Until that moment it had been a very normal, warm summer's day, a week or two before Christmas. I was on call, and the hours had been filled with a medley of farm calls, small animal consults and surgery. I was just locking up the back door of the clinic to go home – I'm sure the on-call gods waited for the last click of the key in the lock – when the after-hours phone rang.

'I need you to come right away! She's bleeding to death!' the farmer cried down the line.

By now I had more than enough on-call work under my belt to understand that there are two sorts of people in an emergency: those who remain calm and, if anything, tend to drastically understate the situation, and those who go to water at the sight of a drop of blood. Mr Elsham was definitely a member of the second group.

Mr Elsham was also one of those rare clients who was unpleasant to deal with. Throughout my career to this point and since, the vast majority of people I've dealt with have been friendly, helpful and, importantly, understanding if things don't go quite to plan. Unfortunately, the exceptions, though they might be few and far between, have a disproportionately negative impact on your mood.

This client had a reputation for micro-managing his employees, and visiting vets received the same treatment. If a single stitch on a wound looked out of alignment, he would point it out, fussing as if this small inconsistency would drastically compromise healing. If our work didn't meet his unrealistically high standards, he was quick to complain to the practice, which meant anyone working with him was always on edge. He hadn't sued over an unexpected outcome yet, but we always felt it was a possibility. And to top all that off, Mr Elsham was well known throughout the northern Victorian dairy industry for his inability to pay accounts on time. Suffice to say he wasn't a favourite client, and a visit to his farm after hours was difficult to be enthusiastic about.

I dragged on my overalls, shoved my feet into my gumboots and drove the 30 minutes to Mr Elsham's farm. As I clambered out of the ute, he rushed towards me, a look of deep concern upon his face.

'There's ... there's blood everywhere,' he stammered. 'Have you got everything for a transfusion?'

'I have everything a large animal vet might need,' I said, keeping my voice steady. 'Now let's examine the patient before we formulate a plan.'

I walked at a brisk but unpanicked pace towards the dairy.

As I suspected, the scene that greeted me at the milking shed was hardly an emergency. Within a crush stood a bright-eyed Jersey cow, a couple of drops of blood on the cement floor underneath her. There was a minute wound visible under her left side, just in front of the udder. I stifled an eye-roll as Mr Elsham came into the shed behind me. This cow certainly did not warrant a blood transfusion. It didn't even need stitches, really. But this was Mr Elsham's farm, so everything had to be done just so.

'If you could ensure her head is properly restrained in the head bail, I'll get a few things together and stitch up the wound,' I said, managing to conjure the appropriate level of enthusiasm.

I returned to the car and pulled out a few ropes, a suture kit and some local anaesthetic. By the time I got back to the shed, Mr Elsham was still struggling to restrain the cow's head in the bail.

'She won't walk forward,' he said, continuing to open and close the bail, seemingly with the idea that eventually the cow would voluntarily stick her head in it. That was unlikely to happen, so I stepped forward, grasped the animal's tail though the side of the crush and waited until he'd opened the bail again. This time, sensing the pressure on her back end, the Jersey obediently walked forward. Mr Elsham closed the bail about her neck.

'There we go,' I said. 'Now if you can hold her tail to distract her while I tie her leg back?'

Mr Elsham took the tail from me and I picked up the ropes to restrain her leg and prevent her from kicking me as I went about my work. I opened one of the side gates for better access, then got the farmer to twitch the tail as I injected some local anaesthetic around the wound, which was only about one centimetre long and looked like it had already sealed itself with a healthy clot. It really didn't need suturing. But for the sake of my own sanity, I would place a stitch – actually, two stitches, to prevent any panic at the possibility of the only stitch failing.

I did the job and stepped back to admire my work. *Nothing to complain about there*, I thought. I undid the ropes and removed them from the back left leg, then closed the crush gate again.

I realised I hadn't drawn up any pain relief for the cow, so I asked Mr Elsham to leave the cow in the crush and returned to the car once more to prepare a syringe. As I stepped back into the dairy, Mr Elsham was hosing down the crush, cleaning the small amount of blood from the side of the cow. I stood beside the crush at the cow's shoulder, then reached over to insert the needle under the skin at the back of the neck.

As soon as the point of my needle touched the skin, the cow kicked out with her back leg in a way that dislodged the latch on the side gate of the crush, causing it to swing open towards me. A bar hit me square in the mouth, and that was when I heard the sound of breaking porcelain.

The pain hadn't hit yet, but the shock was settling in. I ran my finger over my mouth to assess the damage. I felt gaps where they shouldn't have been, and teeth so loose they felt like they were dangling in their sockets. I shuffled to the side of the yard, kneeling down as I felt the blood drain from my head, trying to hold in the nausea and vaguely aware of Mr Elsham fluttering about near me. After a few minutes to regain my senses, I slowly stood up.

I didn't want to speak, as I feared those loose teeth would fall out. Tears rolling down, I tried to make sense of what had happened. I looked at Mr Elsham flapping about and realised that he was possibly in a worse state of shock than I was. There was no way I could trust him to drive me into town to the dentist. Instead, I managed to get myself into the driver's seat of the car, where I called my boss, putting her on speakerphone in the hope that Mr Elsham might at least be able to convey the situation.

'I'be had an accibent,' I said softly, trying to talk through my teeth so as not to disturb them any further.

Why is it that whenever someone asks if you're okay when you're actually not, it causes you to go to water? That's what happens to me anyway. I couldn't respond with words once she asked that question, losing my composure. The tears flooded now.

Mr Elsham tried to babble a response, to which my boss impatiently demanded, 'What has happened to Ameliah?'

I pulled myself together, realising that if I didn't, I'd be wasting a lot of precious time.

'My teeff are shabbered. Cow kick,' was all I could utter between sobs.

'Go straight to the dentist,' he said. 'I'll meet you there to collect the after-hours phone.'

I rang the dentist on my way into Kyabram.

'Hello, this is the dental surgery,' came the friendly voice of the receptionist.

While stifling my tears, I managed to sputter out words to the effect that I was a vet whose teeth had been kicked in by a cow, and that I needed to see the dentist urgently.

The receptionist was so caring it nearly made me cry again. When I got there, the dentist was ready and waiting for me. I will forever be grateful to that dentist, who showed so much compassion for me that evening.

Leaning me back onto the dental chair, she said, 'Don't worry, we've seen much worse.'

She continued to comfort me as she began to assess the extent of damage.

'I'll glue two of them back together. This one,' she said, indicating my right front tooth, 'is too badly shattered. It will need root canal surgery, tonight.'

I nodded my consent and she got to work. It was just on dusk when she completed her temporary repair and told me to come back in the morning. The pain had truly kicked in now, so she sent me home with some pain relief, and wrote me a prescription for something stronger I could get from the chemist the next day.

I thanked them profusely as I left. I felt better, but getting back into the car I went to pieces again. The tears flowed as I started the drive home. I turned the radio on to distract myself and, sure enough, they were going strong on the Christmas songs. The light-hearted jangles turned out to be just what I needed to lift my mood, and as I pulled into the entrance to our house, I found myself joining in to 'All I Want for Christmas is My Two Front Teeth' with a mouthful of cotton wool.

MY BEAUTIFUL WINGS

Early in 2018, life was rolling along pretty nicely. I had a good job, was engaged to a good bloke and, while it wasn't clear when it would happen, I was well on the path to my ultimate goal of becoming a flying vet.

I knew that at some stage I would need to buy my own plane, and had saved some money towards the purpose, but it wasn't something at the front of my mind. I wouldn't need the aircraft until we had concrete plans for returning to our place; there was no rush.

Most of the light aircraft that are currently flown in Australia were originally built in the USA in the 1960s and 1970s. Back then, they were more affordable to buy new, and the exchange rate was a lot more favourable. Planes of this vintage can be bought for around the price of a new four-wheel drive, whereas a newly built plane could cost half a million dollars. But the older planes are perfectly safe – the Civil Aviation Safety Authority (CASA) makes sure of that. Engines are inspected annually and replaced after every 2000 flying hours, propellers are overhauled every ten years, and other components are checked or replaced on a regular basis. As with older cars, the basics are there: they just don't have the bells and whistles of the newer models.

As it turned out, my plane more or less landed in my lap, so to speak.

Every year, my dad and five of his bush pilot mates flew up to Sweers Island in the Gulf of Carpentaria for a fishing holiday. The private island has its own airstrip, so they could fly straight to it. Though Dad has his own plane, their habit was to fly up in two Piper Arrows. These are similar in size to Dad's Cessna 170, but have low wings (that is, the wings spread out from the bottom of the fuselage, not the top), a retractable undercarriage (wheels that fold up into the body after take off, as opposed to being fixed down), and various other features that contribute to making the planes a bit faster than the Cessna. The blokes split themselves between the two aircraft, with the return journey requiring calculations that factored in the extra weight of the catch.

Some time around 2015, one of the crew – Lindsay, an old family friend – managed to buy something he'd always wanted: a twin-engine aircraft. This bigger plane had much longer range than the Arrows and could make the trip from White Cliffs to Sweers in one jump. It was also substantially faster. This was great, but it did leave Lindsay with a quandary.

Since he'd made the upgrade, his little Arrow had sat in the hanger for three years, hardly used. Yet it was still costing him money to keep it flightworthy. Whether a plane is actually flown or not, the compulsory annual mechanical inspection costs a minimum of around $3000, more if substantial servicing is required. Insurance costs around the same.

When I heard about it, I'd told him that I would love to buy it, if only I had the funds. From then on, he would occasionally ring me to ask when I *was* going to buy it. After one of the fishing trips, he told me that he had put his new plane in for a major service and was shocked by the cost of the exercise. He probably shouldn't have been. Most of the focus of a plane's service and inspection is on the engines and propellers. When you have two of each of those instead of one, the cost of that work doubles.

'If you want to get rid of the Arrow and alleviate the financial burden, I can put thirty grand into your bank account tomorrow,' I said. Not for a moment did I expect him to accept this low-ball offer, but I had to get it out there.

'I can't sell it that cheaply,' he said, scoffing.

'That's all I have for now, until I can save some more,' I said.

As I spoke I was doing some quick maths in my head. I'd offered him every cent I had saved, and it would be a while before I had much more to offer. While we are called doctors, average veterinarian earnings are closer to those of allied health professionals like dieticians or physiotherapists than medical doctors. They're okay, but there's not a lot of capacity to save quickly.

We ended our conversation with some light banter, and I figured he'd stew on it and I'd hear from him again in a few months, as usual.

Then, only two weeks later, Lindsay called my bluff. 'If you're serious, it's yours!' he said.

Okay. Now I *really* was going to be broke. But the opportunity was too good to let slip. Before I knew it, I was staring at my empty bank balance on a computer screen, years of savings having magically disappeared into the ether in the way of modern banking.

Cue the *Oh, shit. What have I done?* thoughts. First, I'd just bought an aeroplane that I had yet to actually fly in as a passenger, let alone pilot. Worse, I wasn't even licensed to fly it. The plane had a retractable undercarriage and a constant speed propeller that changed the angle of the propeller blades for optimum efficiency at different stages of flight, especially take off and cruising. So far, I had never flown a plane with these features, and I would need specific endorsements on my licence for both before I could fly it solo.

My other worry related to a saying I'd once heard that anything that starts with an 'f' is better off leased than bought. Something like, 'If it flies, floats or fornicates, it's cheaper and less stressful to hire it.' Well I had just broken that rule. I knew very well that buying a plane, like buying a car, was only the start. The actual purchase is the cheapest part of the journey. I was going to need to keep it fuelled, maintained, and insured.

All of these concerns evaporated into the clear sky above Shepparton Airport on the day I met Lindsay there and first laid eyes on my new bird. He had generously flown her down from his place near ours, in western New South Wales, to deliver her to me. (A lot of aviation language has maritime origins, including the fact that planes, like ships, are all regarded as feminine. I don't know why, but it does seem to suit them.)

I can remember every detail I took in as I ran my eye over her for the first time.

While she was new to me, my aircraft is also much older than I am. Manufactured in the USA in 1969, she's a Piper PA-28 Cherokee Arrow with a 180-horsepower Lycoming engine. Her white paint is flecking off in places, especially on the top of her wings where they have been most exposed to the sun. She has bold red and royal blue stripes down the side that are slightly faded. There's a small luggage door near the tail that gives access to the rear of the cabin. (As I would later learn, it also allows awkward retrieval of your keys if you've locked them inside.) On the side of the cowl (her nose), there is a bronze sign with cursive lettering saying 'Cherokee Arrow', and her call sign is clearly marked on her tail and under her low wings. Her propeller has a simple two blades, grey in colour.

Since I had never even sat in this kind of plane, Lindsay kindly offered to take me up. Even getting in was a novelty – you need to climb up onto the wing and enter through the passenger side, as there is only one door. Once strapped in, we went for a short flight, the old owner in the passenger seat while the new owner (*That would be me*, I kept reminding myself) got the handle of this bird. It was magical, that first flight in a plane that

I *owned*. A thousand times better than the feeling you have when you drive your first car.

'What'll you name her?' Lindsay asked as we parked her up and tied her down.

I looked at her, absorbing all her details again.

'*In a Winna*,' I said.

One day I look forward to giving *In a Winna* a new coat of paint. I often joke that by the time I do that, she won't need sanding back because all the old paint will be gone. But for the moment, practicality is the priority. And anyway, from a distance she still looks neat. And, most importantly, she's mine.

Later that year, I decided that my career needed a shake-up. I had had a wonderful few years in Kyabram, but I wasn't really developing my skills any more. The catalyst for leaving was an opportunity, at the suggestion of a friend, to spend a summer doing locum work in Blenheim, in the Marlborough region at the top of New Zealand's South Island. Leaving Brendan in charge of the animals, I headed off to the land of the long white cloud.

My time working in Blenheim was wondrous. I lived in a charming house at the foot of a mountain on the edge of town, sharing with Rachel, an Irish lass and fellow veterinarian. If you're thinking that having an Aussie girl and an Irish girl living together in one of the world's best wine regions sounds dangerous, you'd be right. We sampled as many wineries as we could on our days off, keeping every empty bottle and building what was ultimately a two-metre-high Christmas tree out of them.

The fresh air and change of scene did wonders for my mood. I returned to Australia with fresh resolve to seriously pursue my lifetime goal: to find a way to go home, set up my practice and start being a flying vet. Thankfully Brendan was fully on board with the idea. He was tired of his work and loved the idea of starting afresh on our big property, and we had enough savings behind us to get started. After another few months of locum work, this time in nearby Tatura, we packed up all our goods and chattels, and animals, and hauled them all 800 kilometres north to the place of my birth.

PART TWO

MY OWN PRACTICE

Returning home in mid-2019 was returning to country gripped by drought. The dry had affected much of Queensland, New South Wales and Victoria since 2017. Vast areas of New South Wales, including much of the western part of the state, experienced their lowest rainfall on record over that three-year period. The conditions brought on by this drought would make a significant contribution to the terrible bushfires experienced down the east coast of Australia in late 2019 and into 2020.

Our home property was faring okay, better than some, though we had weekly dust-storms that were so thick you couldn't see more than five metres ahead on the road. The red dust would creep into every opening it could find: in homes, sheds and vehicles. Our vacuum cleaner got a good workout.

With Dad and Sue still living in the original homestead, Brendan and I moved into what we dubbed the 'cottage'. Standing on metre-high stumps, it's a 20-by-6-metre transportable building, sized just on the maximum allowable to move as a whole without a police escort. It had been built in Adelaide and transported 800 kilometres on the back of a truck. This worked out cheaper than building on site due to the high costs of building material freight and labour in such a remote location. Dad had made the most of Sue's son Nick, a builder by trade, while he and his wife were staying with them for a short while. They had finished off the building between them, with Nick adding a veranda all around and creating a fenced garden.

The cottage sits atop a small sandhill along the airstrip, about 400 metres west of the original house. The old man often jokes that he spread the houses far enough apart that we couldn't throw stones at each other. It's a good distance, though, as both households have privacy. There's an old saying that you should never be able to see your neighbour's clothesline, and we achieve that measure. Across the airstrip we have a view of the lake to the north-east, and it's only a short walk to the hanger and my plane.

Brendan's family, and many of our friends in Victoria, thought that we were mad leaving the green pastures of Victoria for a desolate humpy on the edge of a desert. But while it's true that the Strzelecki Desert is not far away, the existence of the lake creates an oasis where we are.

Of course, it takes planning to ensure we have everything we need out here. There's no running down the street to grab a tub of butter. However, we are well set up with coolrooms and large pantries, so most of the time we want for nothing. On the upside, at least health-wise, we aren't tempted by fast food, and if I conveniently forget to put chocolate or chips on the monthly grocery order, then we have to do without those as well. We have a mail delivery twice a week and most things that you can order online are delivered in reasonable time. I have not been into a clothes shop for years. Mail days can have a vibe like Christmas morning as we unwrap something ordered online but forgotten about while we waited for it. I will never grow weary of that feeling.

One of the benefits of living in isolation is that we only see other people when we choose to. That wouldn't be everyone's cup of tea, but it suits Brendan and me just fine. We get the occasional visit from travelling friends, but mostly, if we feel like socialising, we either meet up with our not-so-nearby neighbours, or travel the hour's drive to the White Cliffs Hotel for a beer and a feed.

The far-west community welcomed us with open arms. Farmers are an aging demographic, and attracting younger people to the bush is getting difficult. Often the maintenance is too much for older farmers to manage on their own. You can see it everywhere: once neat, well-managed farms that have fallen into disarray. Fence lines are overgrown with shrubby weeds, the wire sagging between the posts; ungraded roads are lined with potholes and washouts and barely visible through undergrowth. Woody weeds spread through paddocks once bountiful with native grasslands. It's a real shame to see some of the most beautiful properties become shells of what they once were.

A community needs the energy and enthusiasm, even the idealism, of youth, not only to maintain its physical structure but to keep the community vibrant as well. That's why regions like ours welcome young couples with enthusiasm. More families equates to more community events, more opportunities for sport, more viable shops and more availability of services. With the trend towards greater corporate ownership of properties – there is now as few as one family to every three or so farms – every family makes a difference.

The life we planned at home was always going to combine farming and my vet practice.

On the farm, Brendan and I started out as employees of my dad. This gave Brendan the chance to come to grips with the realities of operating a large property, and me the chance to establish myself as a vet while having an alternative source of income. It also meant I could get back on the farm without buying Dad out, which was something we couldn't afford anyway.

On the vet side, my intention was always to operate a mobile clinic. I had no desire to establish a fully fledged brick-and-mortar clinic or hospital. That would never be viable while living on a remote property anyway, and I had seen enough in other clinics to know that I didn't want the overheads and stress that came with them. Too many vets leave the industry after just a few years, and a lot of that has to do with not finding a way to do what they love – caring for animals – in a way that doesn't physically and mentally drain them. I was determined that this wouldn't happen to me, and that meant doing the sort of work I enjoy most with the types of client I am most comfortable with.

Of course hanging up a shingle to start a business doesn't mean you have customers immediately breaking down your door. The challenges mounted early on, and there were more than a few sleepless nights. Brendan and I had a number of conversations about financial security. What if this mobile vet business idea of mine failed? What if the drought didn't break?

Thankfully, both of us believed that if you spend your life on pause because of all the *what-ifs*, you'll never get anywhere. Brendan had some savings and could always get temporary off-farm work using his fitting and turning qualification. And I could do some locum work, which is what I did.

To begin with, I did a few relief stints for a clinic in Broken Hill that mostly dealt in small animals and animal rescue work. On one occasion, I was asked to take over from the practice's only full-time vet for two weeks while she took a well-overdue break.

I decided to fly down, a trip that would take only about an hour in my aircraft but would have taken three or four by road. Though it costs more to fly, I would have had to drive very early in the day, heightening the risk of coming to grief with a member of the local wildlife as it chose to cross the road at an inopportune moment. When that happens on an outback road at speed, it's always time consuming and expensive, not to mention dangerous. So I justify flying as a form of insurance policy. And of course it is much more enjoyable.

It was around eight in the morning one crystal clear January day when I took to the sky. While mornings are usually the most pleasant time to go flying, the air cool and little or no turbulence, that stillness doesn't last long in the middle of summer in outback New South Wales. When the maximum temperature is headed for 45 degrees, the ground starts to warm within an hour after sunrise. By the time I got to my cruising altitude, the heat was already beginning to rise unevenly from the red earth below, pockets of hot air causing me to bounce around a bit.

After no time at all, Broken Hill and its airport came into view, the town carved into the hill on which it sits. A large wind farm to the north of town dots the hills around Silverton, just before the Mundi Plains. From the air, the white of the wind turbines stand out against their deep-red backdrop. They look enormous, even from the sky.

But there wasn't much time for sightseeing. As with many regional airports, Broken Hill airport doesn't have an air traffic controller. It is the responsibility of pilots to communicate our intentions to each other on an open radio channel and safely navigate clear of each other's flight paths. Ten miles out, I made an inbound call signalling my intention to land. Soon after, a passenger plane from Adelaide made a similar call. They were 20 miles out but travelling faster than me. I radioed back to them to confirm that they'd heard me and check that I was okay to continue my landing ahead of them.

One of the nice things about flying is that old-fashioned airmanship is still the norm. Courtesy and good manners are standard practice in the aviation world. As always there are the occasional exceptions, the pilots who think a bit too much of themselves and, should you meet them on the ground, will tell you how they've done it all and better. But they are rare. One of the customs of this airmanship is that smaller aircraft are allowed to take off and land ahead of larger planes, especially jets. The last thing any small aircraft wants to do is be in a jet's 'wash', the turbulent air blasted out the back of the jet engines. It makes for extremely volatile flying conditions and an horrific experience for the pilot and any passengers.

Communication sorted out, I lined up and made an easy touch down onto the wide asphalt tarmac at Broken Hill. Compared to the dirt tracks I was used to it was like landing on a freeway. As I taxied over to the parking places, I radioed the jet behind me to let them know I was clear of the runway. Then, like parking a very wide car, I selected my spot, pulled in, shut down the engine and removed the key. After climbing out and dragging my bag out of the luggage compartment, I rummaged around to find my tie-down gear and plane cover. I installed these to keep my Arrow in place, should a storm or strong wind gust come through, and protected from the sun in my absence. The heat pillowed up into my face from the tarmac as I did this. It was going to be a scorcher.

I managed to find myself a taxi ahead of the passengers on the Adelaide flight, and within a few minutes was at the clinic and ready for the first of my fortnight's shifts.

'You're early,' said Lottie, one of the nurses, who found me in the smoko room as I clicked the kettle on. I didn't think I was that early until I glanced at the clock on the wall. Once again, I'd forgotten that though Broken Hill is in New South Wales, it runs on South Australian time, which is a half-hour behind the rest of the state. I was close to an hour early after all.

'Oh, well,' I said with a shrug. 'It gives me plenty of time to check the histories and prepare for the day.'

Lottie, a jovial young woman in her early twenties, with short, curly brown hair, laughed. 'You know a walk-in will arrive just on opening time for sure.'

She was almost certainly right. Like the on-call phone ringing just as you nod off, on any day in a clinic when you find yourself with a comfortable amount of time to get organised at the start of the day, an unscheduled patient is sure to arrive and wreak havoc with the schedule.

I made my way around the hospital to see who our patients were and check the handwritten notes on them. The morning nurses and receptionist were busily cleaning out the cages. The usual smells of a vet hospital ward were all there: a potent mix of disinfectant, urine and faeces.

'Has this fella had his pain relief injection yet?' I asked, gesturing towards a labrador lying in a large cage with a drip in his leg.

He had been operated on the previous day to remove a pair of socks he had unwisely considered a meal. Labradors are notorious for foreign body obstructions like this, that require emergency surgery. The socks were double bagged and hanging next to the patient file as a memento for his owners when they came to pick him up. The dog looked rather unimpressed.

'Not yet,' said Mags, another nurse. 'I was waiting for your assessment before we gave it to him.'

I nodded in approval. 'I reckon he could use a half dose this morning. He's feeling a little tense in his abdomen.'

I walked into the drug room and drew the medicine into a syringe, returning to inject it into his drip line.

The rest of the day passed at a rapid pace. After two hours of consults there were three hours of surgery – three scheduled patients and two emergencies. I never did get a chance to make the coffee I'd intended to drink when I arrived, despite reheating the kettle two or three more times in the hope there might be a pause. Lunch was half a sandwich that Mags passed me mid-afternoon, presumably from her own lunch, while I nursed a cat who'd just been operated on for a blocked bladder.

All this is pretty typical for a veterinary clinic servicing the pets of a population of 20,000 people. This clinic had one full-time vet and relied on locums like me to help out in busier periods and when the vet needed a break. That one vet not only worked in the practice during the day, but was on call for evenings and on weekends unless a locum could be found to provide coverage. Despite advertising for years, the clinic hadn't been able to find a second vet and were in a race against time to replace the current vet, who was moving on. While the likes of me try to help out when we can, locums are never going to be a permanent solution. How a vet does it for months on end, constantly overworked and exhausted, is beyond my comprehension.

The same problem exists at vet clinics across rural Australia. It's hard to convince city vets to move out to the bush, and who can blame them? 'Come out west, work 24-7, never get a full night's sleep, have no social life and get paid inadequately for the amount of work you do' isn't a great sales pitch.

Not so long ago, a rural job was the gig all vets wanted. There were usually a number of vets working in one clinic, with everyone sharing the workload and after-hours demands. That had been my experience in Kerang. Today there are more pets, less vets, and owners who demand an ever-higher quality of care. Many vets choose to go out on their own, setting up a mobile service similar to mine, where they can better control their working hours and balance their lives. The pay is the same, but the stress is much lower. We can do our job better because we love it again.

After the first week I was already looking forward to the end of this locum. While I enjoyed being in the clinic with the camaraderie of the nurses and support staff, I was exhausted. I already felt like I was on autopilot, with nothing left to give.

Late in the afternoon at the end of that first week, we were cleaning up the surgery room. I had performed a caesarian section on a bulldog, delivering no less than 11 puppies. They had all survived, though the runt of the litter had taken some effort to revive.

I looked up to see the receptionist, Maddie, shuffling nervously in the doorway.

I raised an impatient eyebrow and Maddie finally said, 'There's a walk-in. A wildlife carer has just picked up an orphaned joey. The mum was hit by a car.'

I nodded, then dropped my head. This day was never going to end.

'I'll be out soon,' I said.

As I forced my aching feet out of the surgery, I noticed an open bag of lollies sitting on the nurses' station. I shoved a handful into my mouth and swallowed them with barely a chew. I could almost feel my glucose levels rising as the sticky mess rolled down my throat, successfully shaking off my grumpiness by the time I got to the waiting room.

'G'day, what little fella have we got here?' I said with a song in my voice. My newfound enthusiasm startled the poor woman who sat there with a pillowcase on her lap. Perhaps I had overdone the sugar.

The woman stood and opened the pillowcase to show me its contents. The infant kangaroo was curled up inside. I put my hand in to feel how cold its skin was, and as I went to touch its back, its little paw came up to meet my hand and curled around my thumb.

And just like that, my heart melted. In an instant my professional don't-get-too-attached-to-the-patient walls were breached.

'She was thrown out and away from mum when the car accident happened. I only happened to notice her in the grass alongside the road after we had been called to clear away the body of the mother,' said the carer.

The joey's paw was quite cool, as was the rest of its body. Cooler than it should be.

'I'm not usually a joey carer,' the woman said after I explained my concerns. 'Margot, who runs the wildlife group, is away for the next few days. I'm not sure what to do until she gets back.'

The carer was visibly relieved when I offered to take the joey into care myself until Margot's return.

And so for the next three days and nights I had a little sidekick. Literally. The best way to keep a little joey warm is with your own body heat, so it lived hanging inside my shirt. I had to hand feed it with a syringe for the first day, until it regained its strength, after which it could suckle a teat from a bottle. While I performed consults and surgeries, the roo hung in its bag on a drip stand in the smoko room. I had a warmed heat pack that I got the nurses to replace often to keep the little fella warm.

By the end of those three days, all the nurses had learnt how to care for a joey. You couldn't get much better practice in preparation for caring for a newborn baby. Getting teenagers to volunteer in an animal rescue nursery might even provide an effective contraception incentive. After a day of feeding a baby kangaroo on the hour, every hour, they might commit themselves to being extra careful.

After Margot returned from her holiday, she came straight in to collect our new friend. Together we examined the joey, taking photos and measuring its weight and the other vitals required for all animals that enter care. Especially in youngsters, it is important to track this information to help judge whether or not the animal is thriving under care. The success of survival in care is directly correlated with weight gain.

The clinic booked the joey in for weekly checks, so as I prepared to return home a few days later, I asked the nurses to keep me posted. Unfortunately, this story doesn't have a happy ending. About a month later the joey was attacked by stray dogs that were roaming the streets of Broken Hill. The carer had pegged the joey in its bag out on the clothesline to enjoy some sunshine on a cool morning. While cleaning up bottles inside, she heard barking and rushed outside to find two dogs jumping and biting at the bag. By the time she had scared them off, the joey was too badly wounded and had passed away.

And that right there is a good example of why we try not to get personally attached to the animals in our care. The difference between empathic care and compassionate care needs to be learnt early on. Empathic care involves placing yourself in the shoes of each individual pet owner or carer, sharing their emotions as though they are your own. When you do this in a role that demands you care for many animals and their owners, it can become very dangerous to your own mental health. Compassionate care allows you to sympathise with your clients while remaining at arm's length emotionally. It's what enables you to conduct your work for the long term in a professional manner. At the risk of sounding harsh, you must detach yourself as much as possible from the emotions that come with the inevitable loss and suffering, otherwise you will certainly break.

Unfortunately this is a distinction that too many in the veterinary profession fail to learn, and it is another contributor to a lot of young vets leaving the profession far too early.

When it comes to rescued native animals, the sad reality is that for every animal that survives to the point of release back into the bush, there are at least two that don't. Some species do better than others, usually because they are less prone to stress. That said, when an animal is released back into the wild, it is a huge moment of achievement and celebration for all involved.

WHELPING DACHSHUND

Slowly but surely the enquiries started to come in and the dream of being a flying vet became a reality – as did the challenge of combining routine farm work with the unpredictable nature of operating an on-call mobile practice.

I had set off to do a bore run one morning, checking the tanks, troughs and bores to ensure our livestock had access to water. That meant also checking the fences and other farm infrastructure along the way; we always keep a coil of soft wire and fence-mending tools in the back of the bore-running ute just in case. Unfortunately, on this day, that kit was missing the all-important leather gloves, so it was just my luck that I'd come across a broken stand of barbed wire. I grunted as I tweaked the replacement barb a click tighter with the fence strainers, beads of sweat rolling down my greasy, heavily sun-screened cheek. By the time I had finished the job, I had plenty of scratches all over the backs of my hands to prove that my morning hadn't been idle. Those gloves would be the first thing back in the ute when I got home.

I'd timed my morning perfectly so that I was finished and back home by smoko time, avoiding the worst of the forecast 49°C on this parched summer's day. Still, the cool house and a cold water guzzled from the fridge were very welcome. I filled the kettle as Brendan and Dad came in from tinkering in the shed, then checked my phone for any calls I'd missed while being out of range in the paddocks. I don't even bother taking my phone out there. My clients understand that I'm not always going to be instantly contactable, many of them being in the same situation.

That morning I had a number of missed calls and a few texts. Of those, one voicemail was more urgent than the rest. I called back, pinning the phone to my ear with my shoulder as I poured coffees for everyone.

'G'day Rach. I got your message. How long since your bitch had the first pup?' I said.

Rachel explained her issue to me while I silently indicated a container of chocolate slice to Brendan. He took that and two cups of coffee out to the porch, where Dad had already lit up a smoke.

The whelping dachshund, Daisy, had delivered one pup several hours ago, but since then no more had arrived. It seemed as though the second puppy was stuck, which meant that Daisy was going to need help.

The challenge was that Rachel was a four-hour drive away from me, near the tiny, remote town of Ivanhoe. She could potentially take the dog to the nearest veterinary hospital, but that was five or six hours away from her, and having Daisy in the car didn't seem wise in her condition. That ruled out meeting me halfway as well. The best option was for me to fly down, which would take me close to an hour and a half by the time I had packed the plane and done my pre-flight safety checks. However that would be a more expensive option for Rachel.

She paused for a minute to think over the options.

'Our strip was used last week by the livestock agent, so it must be okay. If you can fly down that would be great,' she said.

'That settles it,' I said. 'I'll see you soon. I'll send you a text when I clear our runway so you know when to expect me.'

I put my coffee down and hastily gathered everything I might need to deal with the situation, throwing in a piece of fruit for the ride.

'Gotta go,' I said to the men. As I pulled my boots on, I reported which bores I'd checked, smoko being our informal planning time each day.

'What are we going to do with the boss gone?' Dad joked to Brendan as I trudged away.

'Suppose we might just drink coffee for the rest of the day,' said Brendan.

By the time I heard Dad say, 'I'd rather rum and cards,' I was almost out of earshot. I couldn't help wondering whether they would have made the same jokes about my being bossy if I was a bloke. The teasing didn't bother me – I do dislike idleness and I'm well aware that I tend to take charge. It is more the idea that if a woman does that it's bossiness, whereas if a bloke does it's seen as leadership. This is something I've noticed not just in our family but in many family farm businesses in which the women are the ones keeping the ship sailing in the right direction. We might be respected for our contribution, but subtle distinctions like this remain.

Reaching the hangar, I heaved the doors open and loaded my gear into the plane. I inspected the fuel level, then pushed the plane outside for the rest of my checks.

The aircraft was slow to fire up, which I put down to the behaviour of my Arrow in hot weather. Nevertheless, the propeller whirled into action on the second attempt, so I did my run ups and taxied to the far end of the strip. Just as I turned around again, I hit full throttle for a 'rolling take off' – aviation speak for taking off without pausing at the start of the runway. This is customary for bush flying, as keeping moving helps prevent the propeller being chipped by flying gravel.

Being late in the morning on a hot day, this was never going to be a smooth ride. Warm air is less dense, so the plane took a little longer to leave the ground. I retracted the wheels as soon as we cleared the strip, making the plane a little more aerodynamic, but it still felt a touch sluggish. The air rose unevenly in invisible waves from the hot ground, creating plenty of turbulence. Flying at a higher altitude can often reduce this, but even at 6000 feet was pretty unstable on this occasion. These were the sort of conditions that give aerophobic people the jitters.

The country looked dry as I headed south, any glimpses of green pasture now bleached by summer. Below me was a terrain of red earth, pale brown grass and a peppering of grey-green eucalypt foliage.

As I got closer to Ivanhoe, I flicked my UHF radio to Rachel's channel and gave her a call. There was silence for a second, then a crackling reply.

'It's Rachel here.'

'I'm about five minutes away,' I said.

I scanned the landscape in front of the plane's nose, searching for a homestead and nearby airstrip. I soon spotted the silver corrugated roof of a building and, sure enough, just off to the left the distinct clearing of an airstrip, a long, thin patch of cleared, bare red earth. Dust rising from a mob of sheep moving off below gave me an indication of the wind direction on the ground.

I pulled back the throttle and extended the flaps, sinking closer to the ground, then pushed the lever to lower the landing gear. As I did every single time, I let out my breath as the wheels locked into place. One thing about flying an aircraft with retractable wheels is that it's not a matter of *if* but *when* the wheels will get stuck in the up position or not lock down properly. There is an emergency lever which allows you to let them down in a hurry, but it's always comforting to feel the *thunk* of the wheels settling firmly into place.

I turned the aeroplane to line up with the strip. Again I could feel the effects of the warm air, the aircraft descending more quickly and being buffeted about as I approached the ground. Nevertheless, I pulled off a satisfyingly smooth landing.

After stopping mid-runway, I was just pulling the cover over the plane when Rachel pulled up in her Toyota wagon. She was about my age but taller, with tanned skin and the calloused hands of outside work.

'So glad you could come,' she said with a relieved smile. 'Since we spoke, Daisy may have passed another pup, but now she's stuck under the house. I've been trying to get her to come out.'

'The second pup might make my job a little easier, but we'd better get her out,' I said.

Rachel helped carry my gear from the plane to the car and we drove over to the modest house, a transportable building to which, like ours, an all-round veranda had been added to protect the inside from the sun. The house had been placed on raised footings but was only about half a metre off the ground, if that. As I climbed out of the vehicle, I could hear the faint cry of a newborn pup.

Rachel opened the gate of the house-yard and I followed her across the lawn to the edge of the veranda. We both knelt down and peered into the darkness under the house. As my eyes adjusted, I could make out a small burrow smack bang under the middle of the house. Rachel and I shared a knowing look as we both recognised there was no easy way to get there.

'I've got a washing basket with a towel in it we could put the pups in if we can get to them,' Rachel offered.

'That will work well I reckon,' I said, removing my straw hat and sunglasses. 'Maybe grab a lead rope as well, for mum.'

Crawling on all fours, I started to make my way under the house, Rachel following behind me. Swiping away a few spider webs, I was also keeping a wary eye out for snakes as I moved. Dogs aren't the only animals that seek refuge in the cool dark underneath a building.

After making it to the den – really just a shallow hole dug into the earth – I waited for Rachel. I didn't want to disturb the dog, curled up asleep, before her owner arrived. It's always wise to be cautious handling new mums of any species, as hormones can make them extra territorial or protective.

'If you could pat her, attach the lead and coax her out, Rachel, I'll lift the pups into the basket.'

Rachel nodded, reaching down into the den and cooing, 'Now Daisy, it's okay. Come on girl.'

The little dachshund looked up at her owner with a mildly concerned look, then stood up for a pat. We were surprised to see four puppies lying underneath her, and her belly appeared hollow, suggesting there were no more left to come out.

'She's done a great job,' I reassured Rachel as she gently attached the lead rope to Daisy's collar.

With some hesitation about leaving her brood alone, Daisy submitted herself to Rachel's arms. I gingerly lifted each of the tiny pups into the basket, running my eyes over each as I laid them inside. There weren't any apparent abnormalities.

I pushed the basket along in front of me as we crawled our way back out to the lawn, Daisy eagerly following under her own steam. Rachel and I drew in big breaths of fresh air as we emerged, Rachel brushing a handful of spider webs from her blonde ponytail.

One of the pups squeaked for its mother and Daisy jumped into the basket, sniffing and licking each of them, then settling into a comfortable position with the pups nestled along her belly. I checked her vitals with my stethoscope and thermometer – everything looked good – then felt her abdomen. I was fairly confident that there were no more puppies inside, but I wanted to be sure.

'I'll just boot up the scanner to ensure there aren't any left,' I said.

I retrieved my ultrasound machine from Rachel's car, and within a few minutes the screen came alive. I asked Rachel to roll Daisy onto her back and pat her, then applied gel to the bare skin on the dog's underbelly. Sure enough, there were no more puppies to be seen.

'The uterus looks to be shrinking nicely. There's not much fluid in there, so there's little chance of her developing an infection,' I said.

I wiped Daisy's belly clean with a spare towel, cleaned the machine, and packed it away.

'I'm so sorry to have dragged you all this way for nothing,' Rachel said.

'Nah, we couldn't have known how things were going to go. I'd rather come here and have everything turn out well than risk you losing Daisy and her pups.'

'Yes. And it's been much better for me than driving five hours into town.'

Rachel offered me a cold drink before I flew home, which I gratefully accepted. It was going to be another warm, bumpy flight back.

Back at the plane, I was packing my things away when I had a thought.

'Do you have any calcium? To prevent milk fever,' I said.

Milk fever, or canine eclampsia, is a life-threatening condition that comes on suddenly, especially in small dogs. The new mother passes calcium to her puppies through her milk, and if her own calcium level drops as a result, she can become very ill very quickly.

Rachel shook her head.

I pulled a bottle of liquid calcium out of my bag and handed it to her.

'Give Daisy a capful each day until the pups are weaned, which should be at about five weeks old.'

I clambered into the cockpit, which had been kept relatively cool by the plane's cover, now folded and stowed in the luggage compartment.

'I had a little trouble starting the old girl earlier. Would you mind waiting until I've got her going before you drive off?' I said.

'Sure can,' said Rachel.

I followed my usual start-up procedure, but the propeller barely turned over. I repeated the process twice, but still nothing. I cursed myself. It seemed the problem was more than the hot weather, and I had a pretty good idea that it was either a dodgy starter or, more likely, a flat battery.

I have a history of battery issues in cars and planes. My frugality is something of a running joke within my family, and batteries are a good example. *You don't get money by spending it all* is my thinking, flawed though that may be at times. During my university days I once jumpstarted my old Ford Falcon ute all the way from Toowoomba to home because a set of jumper leads was cheaper than a new battery. A car full of Aboriginal boys gave me a push start at the Bourke petrol station in a scene straight out of the old TV show *Bush Mechanics*. Now my tight-arse tendencies had come back to bite me again, this time with my plane. I'd known the battery was getting on a bit, but chose to repeatedly recharge the old one rather than fork out for a new one.

I unclipped my belt and climbed out. Some confident pilots can start a plane by spinning the propeller over by hand – 'prop starting' – but that wasn't an option for me. I didn't have the strength to pull the prop around, nor the agility to jump out of the way when it did fire up.

'I think I need a jump start,' I called to Rachel in her car.

Rachel drove over and pulled up next to the plane. I popped open the bonnet and we hooked a pair of jumper leads up in the same way you do with a car. Thankfully the aircraft's battery was easily accessible behind the luggage door.

'Okay. When I get her going, please disconnect the leads from the plane,' I said.

I hopped back into the cockpit, and this time the engine sparked to life first time.

I left the plane idling while I got out to disconnect the leads at my end. I could immediately smell burning plastic, and Rachel stood in front of her car holding a pair of semi-molten clamps.

'I was a bit slow pulling these off,' she said, staring at the now misshapen ends.

'I should have warned you,' I said. 'The plane sucks a fair bit of current when it starts up.'

I replaced the cover of the battery, cursing with shock as I accidentally touched the spanner connected to a terminal, firing off a large spark. No harm done, other than a rush of adrenalin and a few minutes of elevated heart rate.

I shook hands with Rachel.

'Thanks for the jump start. Sorry about the leads.'

Rachel laughed.

'I've learnt something about jump starting a plane today,' she said.

I smirked. 'So have I.'

CASTRATING PODDY

'**G**'day Doctor,' said the gruff voice over the phone. 'I hear you do large animals.'

The voice went on to introduce himself as Harry, from a cattle station between Ivanhoe and Wilcannia.

'I do,' I replied. 'Livestock and horses are my special interest.'

'Well, I've got a few head for you to have a look at.'

When farmers say they have a 'few', I know to expect any number between five and 2000.

'Too easy. How many head, and what do you need done?'

'I got a good deal on some weaners from Western Australia. 800 head of shorthorn heifers and steers.'

Turned out Harry's 'few' was at the higher end!

'They got here about four months ago,' he continued, 'and they don't seem to have picked up as quickly as I'd expected'.

I took a second to process this. It's quite normal for young cattle, transported such a distance and now feeding on different pastures, to take some time to adjust before putting on weight. But I'd need to see them to confirm whether or not there was something else at play. I arranged to fly down the following week to examine them, confirming as usual that his airstrip was serviceable.

'Oh, and one other thing,' Harry said, just before we ended the call. 'I've got a bull that needs castrating. I'd normally do it myself, but I've been feeding him through the drought so he's become my pet.' He sounded embarrassed at having to ask.

'Of course I can do that for you,' I said. 'I find it hard to treat my own pets. It's difficult when you've got an emotional attachment.'

A few days later I practically skipped down to the hangar. The morning was absolutely perfect for flying: cool, clear and still. There's nothing better than flying through the silky air in conditions like this. As I pushed open the hangar doors, the first rays of sunlight trickled in to reveal my lovely plane waiting for me, fuelled up and packed the night before. I collected the hand steer tool and attached it to the front wheel. The tool helps me keep the plane straight as I push her backwards out of the shed.

Checks done and ready to go, I turned the key to fire up the Arrow's engine. There was a groan, but no action. I tried again, then again, and on that third attempt the prop finally spun into action.

Bloody battery. Must do something about that, I thought to myself … again.

After the episode at Rachel's I always made sure I had my own set of jumper leads in the plane's toolkit. If worse came to worst, I could get Harry to give me a jump start this afternoon to get home. I'd conveniently kicked the can of the more obvious solution down the road. I would buy a new battery eventually.

I turned at the end of the strip, pushed the throttle all the way in and raced down the runway. Extending the flaps a little – flaps can assist with take off as well as landing – the wheels lifted from the ground. As soon as we were clear, I retracted the flaps and pulled the gear lever up, tucking the wheels inside the plane and immediately feeling the increase in power with the reduction in air drag. Lovely.

Today's flight was only 40 minutes, but it saved me over two hours in each direction compared with driving. Flying does feel quick, though. I'd barely reached my cruise altitude of 3000 feet before beginning the descent. While it was still early, there was already a bit of turbulence as I got closer to the ground. It was going to be another warm day. I know many people cannot stand the sensation of turbulence, but to me it's like riding waves on a boat – only the waves are invisible.

Harry had told me he had a dirt strip, and said he would have it freshly dragged to ensure it was smooth. This made it easy to find as well, a lighter red strip clearly standing out from the richer red surroundings. The strip was marked with white-painted tyres along its edges. Dust rising from what must have been Harry driving towards the strip indicated the wind direction to me. Landing into the wind, the airstrip was a little bumpy but safe enough for the plane.

Harry's old white Nissan Patrol ute, with its inevitable dents from nocturnal wildlife collisions, arrived just as I pulled my vet box out of the luggage compartment. I shook hands with him through the window. He looked tall, probably mid-sixties, with weather-beaten tanned skin. He wore an old truck cap, navy shirt with ripped pockets and well-worn jeans. This man looked like he knew how to work.

'Jump in,' he said. 'I'll take you around the main mob and then to the cattle yards. I've got 100 of them yarded for you to get a closer look at.'

The paddock the cattle were in was large, around 5000 hectares (12,000 acres), and full of drying Mitchell grass – the most common form of native grass in the region and good cattle pasture – and herbage. The cattle I could see were spread out along the creek bed that ran through the middle of the field. They were small-framed shorthorns with a healthy shine to their coats, although they did appear to be light in condition. As we got closer, I could see that none of them had any discharge from their noses and their back ends were clean, which ruled out diarrhoea.

As we drove around the paddock, we chatted about their history and treatments that he'd given them so far. They were up-to-date with vaccinations and had been drenched for worms after arriving from the west.

At the yards about an hour later, I walked through the mob. Like their mates out in the pasture, they had a healthy shine and no outward signs of illness, though again they were skinny.

'Could we draft out ten of the slimmest ones?' I said. 'I'll give them a closer examination in the crush.'

They were well-handled, quiet cattle, easy to look over. I took a faecal sample from each to discount the possibility of a worm or gastrointestinal issue. I would test the samples when I got home.

'I'll let you know if I find anything, but I doubt it. I think it's just the big change they've gone through. They were weaned early, then had that long voyage across the country. They most likely just need a little more time to catch up.'

Harry nodded. 'Fair enough. It's good to know there's nothing wrong,' he said.

It can be challenging sometimes when you make a trip out to a new client like this and the best thing to do is nothing. There's always the temptation to find *something* that needs to be done, even if it's token, to justify the journey. But in this case, confirmation that all was okay was all I could reasonably offer. Harry seemed satisfied with that.

'Could you have a look at my poddy?' said Harry.

'Sure thing,' I said, looking about the yard for a little bull.

'He's down in the back yard. I'll bring him up into the crush.'

As Harry made his way through the mob of weaners, I could make out a large figure at the back of the yards. It was no poddy calf. This fully grown bull, which Harry *called* Poddy, was gigantic. Triple the size of the rest of the cattle. No wonder he was a way off on his own. He'd do some damage if he got into a scuffle with a smaller beast.

A few minutes later the large, red-coated bull – I thought most likely a Droughtmaster, an Australian breed originally from Queensland – loped down the race. He obediently stopped in the crush for his turn with the vet. Harry came up behind him, giving him a scratch on the rump as he closed the crush gate behind. The bull relaxed his left leg into the scratch, then gave Harry a pleading look when he stopped his attentions. This was a heck of a big pet.

'His mum didn't survive the worst of the dry and I found him at a bore on his own when he was only a few days old,' said Harry. 'That's when I named him Poddy. If it wasn't for this fella, I probably wouldn't be here myself. I struggled to keep going some days, but on those days when I was slow to get myself out of bed, I'd hear him bellowing out for his breakfast and had to get up to feed him.'

I gave him an understanding smile. Depression rates skyrocket within the agricultural industry during times of drought. It's very difficult to detach yourself from your livelihood when you live where you work, and when you see animals starving to death and aren't able to help them, it weighs down on you.

It's a problem that has been exacerbated in the bush for decades, due to the peculiarly Australian taboo, amongst men especially, on discussing how they're feeling. The suicide rate amongst farmers has been reported at 60 per cent higher than non-farmers. Thankfully there is an increasing awareness about depression and mental health services are becoming more available to farmers, but there's still room for improvement, and a long way to go.

In the meantime, service-providing professionals, such as myself, are the only outside contact many farmers have away from their social circles. They often find it easier to talk to us – as 'outsiders' – about their struggles than they can to their families or mates. Often, they don't want to impose any extra burden on the people close to them. Nevertheless, it is often a family member who first seeks help for a loved one dealing with the black dog, which of course can't happen if you live on your own. That's where having a hobby or an interest that pulls you physically and mentally away from your struggles can be key to clearing the haze of sadness. Luckily for Harry, this bull had been the commitment he needed to keep him going each day.

'I can't bear to see him in any pain,' he said now.

'He will be two stone less, without any pain. I'll give him a sedative and some local anaesthetic and he won't have a clue what I'm doing back here.'

When I stepped in behind the animal, the top of his tail was above my head. His big cojones swung between his legs, reaching down to his knees. Each testicle was the size of a football. I gulped. One kick from this fellow and I was a goner! I gently inserted the sedative needle into the vein underneath his tail, letting out a sigh of relief when I removed the syringe and there were no objections. I then drew up a large syringe of local anaesthetic. Once the bull had lowered his head, I knew the sedation had taken effect and he was feeling relaxed.

Now I got Harry to hold the tail in a tight twist to distract the bull while I injected the local into the scrotum. Given his size, I had to draw up several lots of anaesthetic to adequately numb each gonad. The bull twitched his ears as I inserted the needle, but that was all he did in protest.

After testing the back of the scrotum by poking it with the tip of a needle, I was satisfied that my pain block had been successful. I readied for surgery, laying out my kit on top of a 44-gallon drum Harry had placed beside the side gate of the crush. No sterile operating theatres out here. After I'd given the scrotum a good clean with disinfectant, Harry held the tail away to the side as I made my incision with the scalpel. I used emasculators to clamp the spermatic cord attaching each testicle, then cut the testicles away. After unclamping the emasculators, I was pleased to see there was no bleeding from the scrotum.

Not expecting such a large animal – most castrations are done on much younger bulls – I hadn't planned on the large amount of loose scrotal skin that remained. I didn't like the look of it, dangling between his legs.

'I'm going to remove that skin and suture the scrotum closed,' I explained. 'Normally I'd leave it to heal in an open manner, but he has a lot of spare skin here.'

It only took a few quick cuts to remove the scrotum, leaving enough skin in his groin to suture together. I used dissolvable stitches, not wanting anyone to mess about removing sutures from this mammoth in a few weeks if it could be avoided. After the skin was cleaned up with a few splashes of clean water, I stepped back to assess the surgery wound. It looked good.

I asked Harry to let go of the tail, then opened the front of the crush for the big fellow to move out, which he did with a few wobbly steps.

'He's still got the sedation on board. He'll be back to normal in about an hour,' I said. 'Keep him in the yards for two weeks, away from females.'

'Ah yes, we don't want all our hard work ruined by Poddy getting randy with a heifer,' said Harry.

'A lesson many young blokes could learn, eh?" I laughed.

Harry responded with a roguish smile. 'Old blokes need to be reminded too. Some think a fine tune can be played on an old fiddle, but these days, my fiddle only works once a week.'

I couldn't help but chuckle at that. 'As long as you've got a few tunes left in you, that's the main thing.'

One of the reasons why I love being out in the middle of the sticks is the dry sense of humour that thrives in the bush. Without a sense of humour, life out here would be so much tougher. Humour is how many people get through the hard times; it develops from those times of strain. It's like a shield that protects us from the harshness of outback life.

'Cup of tea?' Harry offered as we climbed into his ute.

'That'd be lovely' I said.

We drove to the homestead, a small weatherboard house surrounded by a waist-high netting fence to keep cattle from eating the lawn. I removed my boots and hat at the front door and sat down at the kitchen table. The house was neat for a bachelor pad. We chatted about family and our lives. Harry had two sisters who often visited with their children in the school holidays.

'I never had kids of my own, but one of my nieces is keen on farming,' he said. 'She reckons she's coming out here when she finishes school next year.'

There was a glint in his eyes as he said this. He was looking forward to having some company. But he also reflected the widespread desire to see younger people in the bush. Harry saw the potential benefits to the farm and the community of having his niece around.

We finished our cups of tea and Harry drove me back to the airstrip. It was early afternoon by now and the heat was radiating off the red sand.

Thankfully the engine turned over first time. As I cleared the runway the plane bumped around until I reached smooth, cool air at about 5000 feet. On the journey home I thought more about

Harry, about how lucky it was that he was able to negotiate the hardship of drought and depression on his own. I knew very well that this wasn't always possible. Too many farmers found themselves unable to see their way through the fog of sadness and loneliness. It reminded me of the importance of maintaining social connections, even when we are all separated by hundreds of kilometres.

ON THE ROAD
AGAIN ... AND AGAIN

One of the obvious challenges of being a mobile vet, and the only vet, covering a vast territory – a territory almost the size of England – are the logistics.

As much as I would love to spend all my time in the plane, it just isn't practical to fly when I need to see a number of clients across a string of small towns. Apart from the fact that I'd be taking off and landing almost more than flying straight and level, the weight limitations of the aircraft prevent me carrying the wide range of medications and equipment I need to properly service every community I visit.

Then there are all the properties that don't have a serviceable airstrip. 'It's got a few potholes,' is a common answer to my question about the condition of a farm's runway, which is a euphemism for 'bloody rough and best not used except in an emergency'.

After a fair bit of trial and error, I discovered that a monthly road trip, in a loop-like fashion around the far west, works best for providing a regular service. My dual-cab four-wheel-drive ute, heavily equipped and fully stocked, makes the trip as comfortable and as efficient as I could hope for. I use my plane for jobs that don't require bulky equipment or that are remote or far enough away that air travel works better. As a rule of thumb, anywhere more than an hour's drive from home is a candidate for a flight if it's a one-off job.

The typical road trip takes a full seven-day week and covers around 3500 kilometres, averaging about six hours driving per day. I visit the communities around White Cliffs, Wilcannia, Ivanhoe, Balranald, Pooncarie, Menindee, Packsaddle, Tibooburra, Wanaaring, Louth and Tilpa. Look at a map and you'll notice that all these places sit in a large rectangle bordered roughly by the Barrier Highway in the south, Kidman Way in the east, and the South Australian and Queensland borders in the west and north. It's an area of around 135,000 square kilometres. During these trips, I see everything from cats, dogs and other small domestic animals to horses, cattle, sheep, goats, alpacas, and even camels. Along the way, I spend time with a lot of lovely people and plenty of bush characters with personalities carved out of the environment in which we all thrive.

My ute is well stocked under its custom canopy, complete with an upright fridge and stainless steel drawers stocked neatly with all the medications and provisions I am likely to need. I carry my portable X-ray and ultrasound machines, anaesthetic machine, oxygen generator, otoscope (for ear inspection, very similar to the ones human doctors use), PowerFloat (for equine dentistry) and laptop. A lot of this I was able to buy second hand, thanks to the generosity of a number of my peers. The two things I bought new were the anaesthetic machine and the oxygen generator, the latter of which saves me from carrying dangerously explosive oxygen bottles around with me. The car has bright spotlight high beams attached to the bull bar at the front, which are especially useful during winter when it's hard to fit an entire workday into the fewer hours of daylight.

Before I head off on a road trip, all battery-operated equipment, such as my clippers and the PowerFloat, is fully charged. I make sure my phone has plenty of music and podcasts downloaded to keep me entertained during the hours of driving.

I wake at five o'clock on the first morning of the circuit, the world still dark, and make a coffee and toasted sandwich for the road. After sneaking into our bedroom to give my still-slumbering husband a goodbye cuddle, I head off. Often the sun pops up just as I turn out of our 15-kilometres driveway and onto the gravel main road. So it will be each day for the rest of the week, the sun appearing as I drive to my first client and disappearing as I finish the last.

A typical day on the road starts with the rude blaring of the alarm jolting me from my slumber in a small hotel room in a small country town. I clamber into my clothes, carefully laid out the night before, pour coffee into my travel mug, jump into the car and, as the sky lights up, head to my first appointment.

The town in question might be Menindee, 100 kilometres south-east of Broken Hill, where I'll spend the day attending to the pets of the townsfolk. The outback town has a population of only 600, though it has two pubs, two cafés, a supermarket, a service station and a chemist. It's a town where the children walk or cycle to school from their weatherboard or tin-clad cottage-style homes, and where most of the working population relies on agricultural industries.

On this typical day, I'll have a multitude of household pets to vaccinate, toenails to trim, worming tablets to administer and the odd anal gland to squeeze. Anal glands in dogs, cats and some other mammals sit just under the skin adjacent to the anus. They produce a smelly fluid that gives the animal's faeces, and its bottom, a unique fragrance. It's because of these glands that dogs 'introduce' themselves by smelling each other's bottoms, and why they take so much interest in any poo they come across in the street or park. Occasionally the anal glands can get clogged up, which causes discomfort in the animal and can lead to infection and worse. The way to remedy this situation is for the lucky vet to insert a gloved finger into the rectum and massage and squeeze the glands to free them up. It is not the most pleasant of procedures, not least because of the fairly malicious odours that can be emitted from an anal gland, and particularly a blocked one.

One day, I was in the middle of this exercise with the fox terrier belonging to John, one of my clients, when he asked an unusual question.

'Why do animals try to hump people?'

John was in his 40s, his Greek heritage reflected in his solid build, dark hair and olive skin. He was a jovial man, always making light of life, though his expression this time was a bit more earnest. I realised he wasn't joking.

I removed my finger from the dog's rectum, pulling my gloves off and promptly disposing of them and their stench.

'There are many causes for inappropriate behaviour in animals. Sometimes it can be lack of socialisation. Sometimes they can be in season, with a strong urge to mate, and if they lack an appropriate mate, they try to make do with substitutes,' I explained.

John took this on board but continued to shuffle uncomfortably on the spot.

'I think our pet goat might have some issues. Last week he began exhibiting himself to the postie.'

I gave John a rueful smile as he described the goat's antics. Mr Stinky the billy goat would rear up on his hindlegs as the postman approached, with his 'old Roger' fully extended.

'He even makes a different bleat when the postie is coming, like he's calling out to a lover. It's a long, melodious *baaa*. The poor old postie has to keep clear of the fence to avoid being, well, sprayed, due to Mr Stinky's overexcitement.'

By this stage of John's yarn I was laughing so hard I had tears rolling down my cheeks.

'Now it's gotten worse,' he went on. 'He's started doing it to everyone who passes by. We've had to lock him out the back so he can't harass passing children.'

After regaining my composure, I asked whether or not the goat had been castrated.

'Ah, no. We weren't sure how to go about it. Can you put a ring on them like a lamb?' John said.

'If he's younger than six months old you can, but if he's older, it has to be done by a vet,' I said.

'He's about 10 months old now. Would you have time to look at him?'

I was only too happy to oblige. John showed me down to the backyard, where the goat had a pen in the far corner under a large gum tree. He had a shaggy coat of grey fur and an impressive set of horns that had grown to span almost a metre straight out from his wide head, with a slight upward twist at the tips.

Mr Stinky lived up to his name. I could smell the strong aroma produced by his pheromone glands, which I imagined must smell like sweet jasmine to a female nanny goat, though definitely not to a human. He stood with his front feet up on the panels of the fence, his penis erect, gyrating up and down while his large testicles swung gaily between his hindlegs. This is the caprine method for self-pleasure. I was impressed at how he managed to continuously secrete fluid as he rocked to and fro upon the panel.

I cleared my throat. 'I think we had better do something about this sooner rather than later. I'll castrate him today, if you're happy for me to proceed?'

'Thank you,' said John, visibly relaxing at the idea. 'I was worried that I might be reported to the police for having a public nuisance.'

I tried in vain to stifle a smirk.

'I'll need a 10-litre bucket of clean, clear water,' I said. 'And I need to collect a few things from the car. I'll be back in five.'

At the vehicle, I pulled out my surgery box and gathered some sedatives. I'd learnt from past experience with goats that they can be very vocal when being manhandled. During my time in Victoria I'd had an old pet goat as a patient. He had bad arthritis that was managed for several years with pain medication, but when it became ineffective the owner opted to have him euthanised. I went out to the home at the end of the day, taking a fellow vet to help as the owner didn't want to be present for the procedure.

When we arrived, the whole extended family was there saying their last goodbyes. They all went around to the front of the house and left us to do our part. As I touched the point of the catheter to the skin of the jugular vein, the goat began to bleat. In an effort to quieten the animal, my comrade placed a hand over his eyes, but this only made things worse. The goat panicked and began to scream. I pressed on with trying to place the catheter into the vein, but every tiny movement only escalated the goat's cries. Panicking at the shrieks, my comrade covered the animal's mouth to muffle them, upon which the goat let out a blood-curdling scream that could have shattered glass.

By now our ears were ringing and I was certain the family on the other side of the house would be wondering what was going on. The 'good death' we vets claim to be able to deliver was not happening with this patient. Finally I chose to race back to the clinic and get some sedation, which we then administered before injecting the final euthanasia drugs. For a long time after that my colleagues in the clinic dubbed me the 'goat murderer', and memories of the racket still make me cringe.

It was with that old goat in mind that I drew up a decent dose of sedation for Mr Stinky, enough to guarantee there would not be any glass-shattering screams from this patient. I placed the capped syringe into my front shirt pocket, picked up my surgery box and strode back to my patient. Showing confidence is key in a situation like this. Any faltering in resolve will be sensed by an animal, particularly a goat. They have an uncanny knack of knowing when your guard is down.

John had set a bucket of water next to the gate of the pen and was leaning on the gate waiting for me. He turned to me as I set down my implements next to the bucket.

'I reckon it'll take both of us to catch him,' he said as he opened the gate and stood aside to allow me through. 'Ladies first!'

I smiled in thanks and entered the pen. When Mr Stinky, somewhat calmer now, casually walked up to me, I offered an outstretched hand. He sniffed and attempted to nibble my fingertips, me curling my hand into a tight ball to discourage him from taking a bite. All of a sudden, before I could blink, he was on top of me. He leapt up onto my chest, knocking me backwards and into John, who was behind me.

Fortunately, John broke my fall, holding me up with his hands on my back, but Mr Stinky meant business. Once again he was rocking back and forth on his back legs with his penis extended, but this time it was my shoulders he was leaning on, not the fence. I swatted at the serial pest, trying to push him away, but he stood firmly, with his front feet upon either side of my chest, effectively pinning my arms to my side.

'I'll get him,' John said, and as he stepped forward, I stepped to the side. John grabbed Mr Stinky by the horns, which gave me time to move away. I fumbled into my shirt pocket, found the syringe, yanked the cap off the needle. While John continued to hold the goat steady, I stepped around him and jabbed the sedative into the animal's rump. He let out an almighty shriek of objection.

'It will take about five minutes for that to take effect,' I said. 'We'll need to hold him still until it does.'

Mr Stinky dropped back onto all fours while John and I each held one of the goat's horns, keeping him headlocked. We both let out audible sighs as he began to wobble, the effects of sedation beginning to show. Finally the animal sat back on his haunches, before lying down like a lamb at our feet. John and I exchanged smiles of relief.

I tentatively brushed Mr Stinky's right ear to test how drowsy he was. There was no reaction, his ear flopping back in place.

'He's out for the count,' I affirmed, more to myself than anyone else.

I collected the gear from outside the pen and set it down behind the tail end of the goat. Pulling my hair clippers from the box, I hummed to myself as I set about preparing the area for surgery. After removing the fur from the back of the scrotum, I washed the skin with antiseptic and put on my gloves. It only took 30 seconds to remove both testicles.

'I'll leave these incisions open for drainage,' I said, double-checking for any bleeding. 'Make sure he moves about, as that will help keep the swelling down.'

I drew up a large syringe of long-acting penicillin and injected it into the rump muscle, then followed that with a dose of pain relief administered under the skin over the shoulders. Mr Stinky began to move slightly, the sedation already wearing off. Observing his recovery as I cleaned up my hands and surgical equipment in the bucket of water, I saw Mr Stinky lift his head while remaining seated. He looked back over himself, as if he were assessing what had happened. He then looked back at me and gave a long, low wail.

'I reckon he's telling you just how upset he is at losing his crown jewels!' said John.

'Seems to me he had it coming. He couldn't assault me like he did and expect to keep them,' I said.

John laughed in agreement.

'He'll be standing within the hour,' I said as I shook John's hand. 'Any issues, you know how to get me.'

I packed up my car, reflecting that I still had a thing or two to learn about dealing with randy goats. As always, each experience helps prepare you better for the next.

I made my way to the next job, where the first thing the next client said was, 'Gosh, you stink!'

WILD HORSES AND
ACCIDENTAL SURGERY

'Have you got a dart gun?' asked the farmer over the phone. He'd introduced himself as Rodney, and told me he was on a station near Pooncarie, a village on the Darling River, 150 kilometres from Mildura.

I rolled my eyes. The number of times I've been asked this! I blame various television shows that dramatise vets using dart guns to sedate or capture wild and feral animals. Now everyone thinks vets run around shooting darts at any animal – domestic or wild – that's large enough to be a potential source of danger.

The perhaps boring reality is that the priority with all animals is to handle them appropriately and safely, in a way that won't require the intervention of drugs. In the case of domestic animals, it is far less stressful for both human and beast if they become used to human interaction.

Wildlife is another matter, where human interaction is to be avoided and, occasionally, a dart gun will be needed to restrain an animal prior to, say, treatment or relocation. But even with wildlife, sedation isn't universally used. In the rare instance that I'm called to look after a wild animal, the sick or injured animal is already in the hands of a registered wildlife carer and used to being near humans. No dart gun needed.

What many people don't realise is that the sedation required for darting wild animals is extremely dangerous. One scratch into a person's skin would be enough to kill. The drugs behave differently in humans than animals, so when using them for dart guns, an antidote is kept at the ready with a letter of instructions for anyone nearby to inject it. There is a real risk when accidentally self-injected that you will pass out before you can administer the antidote to yourself. But even with animals, a tranquilliser shot via dart gun is inherently more dangerous than one administered by injection. The dart not only has to hit the animal, but hit the right spot to be effective. Many vets will agree, there is enough danger involved in our line of work without adding highly lethal drugs to the mix.

I conveyed all this to Rodney. For some reason I'd formed the impression that this bloke was asking about darting in relation to rounding up wild cattle he figured he could capture and sell, so I went on to explain that darting wild cattle (also known as 'scrubber bulls' or 'mickeys') is not an option, as animals caught that way would need to be kept for six weeks prior to slaughter. If he tried to sell them before that period and any trace of the drugs was found in the beast, the whole animal would be condemned at the abattoir and his effort would have been for nothing.

However, it turned out I'd read him wrong.

'Ah, no, Doc,' Rodney said. 'It's not cattle I'm askin' about. I got me some stallions. They are nice-lookin' fellas and well-bred. I want to keep them as pets, not have them become wild and end up being sent to the knackery. Me daughter was meant to get them quiet, but she started havin' kids, and now they're too big and full of themselves for me to handle on me own.'

'Oh,' I said. 'That I might be able to help you out with. How old are they, and how tall? And how many?'

'There are five of them, paints and quarter horses, about 15 hands I reckon.'

'Have they had any handling at all?' I said.

Rodney sounded a little embarrassed as he responded. 'Ah, not much. I can pat them on the head and neck, but I can't run my hand underneath the belly on any of 'em.'

Jeez, I thought. *They're going to be a handful.*

'I was hoping they might calm down without their knackers,' Rodney added.

'That would certainly help to calm them down,' I agreed. Preventing testosterone coursing through their veins would have that effect. 'But in order for me to castrate them, I need to be able to put a stethoscope on their chest and insert a needle into their neck to sedate them. Using a dart isn't an option in a case like this, for all the reasons I explained earlier.'

'I reckon I could get halters on 'em, but I might need some time to do that before I get you to come,' he admitted.

We ended the phone conversation with him agreeing to book the castrations for when he had them more tamed.

A month went by before I heard from Rodney again.

'I got 'em all in halters. I can pet them up under their shoulders and they don't mind it when I pinch them on the neck,' he reported.

'No dramas,' I said. 'I'm going to be coming through your area next Monday in the car. I'll drop in first thing, and we'll see if I can take the cheek out of them.'

Although I still had my doubts, I took him at his word that the horses were able to be safely handled. I grinned to myself as I hung up the phone. This was going to be an interesting experience.

I drove down the dirt road to Rodney's homestead, the soil the typical rich black colour of this country along the Darling. My ute sent up clouds of black dust as the road wound amongst a dense clump of mallee gums. There was little grass around, this area also suffering the effects of drought.

As I rounded another bend of the river, I could make out some yards ahead. Rodney had told me that the horse yards were before the house, so he would meet me there. They were constructed of reasonably new galvanised panels, the steel glinting against the dark gum-tree forest. Within the pens I could make out several large horses. I was in the right place. It was a lovely tranquil spot, right on a bend of the Darling, underneath the mallee trees.

As I pulled up at the yards, I could see more dust clouds heading my way from the opposite side. Rodney was on his way.

I stepped out to inspect the horses, which were in separate pens on the edge of the plain round yard. Each yard had a soft, sandy floor, perfect for horses to lie on, and each animal had on a halter with a short lead rope hanging down off the chin strap. They all appeared relaxed and in good body condition, with the thick, muscular necks characteristic of stallions.

Rodney's old Triton ute rounded a bend, rattled and bumped over a few potholes and came to a stop beside my car. The door creaked as he got out and it needed a forceful slam to shut. At that the horses' heads all jolted up, their nostrils flaring. Perhaps they weren't as quiet as I'd thought.

Rodney was a short man, his head at my shoulders. I figured he was probably in his seventies, with a thick mat of short, uncombed grey hair stuffed underneath an old sheep-cocky's felt hat. He was wearing a flannel shirt and jeans, ready for work.

'Good of you to come,' he said as we shook hands. 'I've got a few buckets of clean water and a heap of towels, just as ya asked me.'

'Righto,' I said, removing my stethoscope and a vial of sedative from the stainless steel drawers in the canopy of my ute.

I started to draw a dose of sedative into a syringe.

'If you'd like to catch the first patient, I'll check him out and sedate him.'

Rodney opened the gate of the round yard and walked across to the closest pen on the right, which contained a bay stallion. As the farmer entered the pen, closing the gate behind him, the horse backed into the farthest corner. He held his head high as he eyed the intruder. Waiting at the entrance to the round yard, I chewed my lip with concern. Hopefully with some petting and slow movements I might be able to get the horse sedated safely.

Rodney approached the horse slowly, taking the lead rope into his hands then giving it a gentle pull to encourage the animal forward. The stallion thought for a moment, then cooperated. Once he had taken a couple of steps and was standing in the middle of the pen, I made my way over, careful in my movements so as not to startle him.

The other stallions looked at me with interest as I approached. I quietly opened the pen's gate, leaving it open this time in case we needed to escape the confined space. Again the horse raised his head, nostrils flaring, so I stood still for several minutes, cooing to reassure him. Finally he dropped his head and leaned his nose forward, sniffing towards me. I eased myself towards him, extending my arm for him to sniff. Introduction made, I patted his face, down his neck and across his shoulders. He was understandably a little apprehensive – other than Rodney I was the first human he'd had any contact with in a long time – but he remained calm.

After a few more moments stroking his shoulders and chest, I placed the stethoscope into my ears and gently laid it upon the side of his chest. He danced on the spot as the oddly-shaped tool touched his fur. His heart sounded fine though, and I was satisfied the sedation would be safe.

I looked about the pen as I pulled the syringe from my pocket. It was only three metres wide. If the horse felt threatened by my needle in this confined space he could do himself or us a serious injury, so I suggested to Rodney that he lead the animal into the middle of the circular yard. With the stallion standing there, I approached him once again and stroked his neck. I eyed Rodney, who was standing in front of the horse with his left hand loosely grasping the side strap of the halter, near the animal's face.

'I don't think you should stand like that for what I'm about to do,' I said. 'When I insert this needle, he will probably jump either forward or backward. It would be best if you stand to the side with me. And hold the lead rope, not the halter.'

'I'll be right,' he said. 'I've handled horses since before you were born.'

He kept his grasp on the halter, but he did shuffle more to the side. I frowned, but decided not to press the issue any further. He had been warned.

I uncapped the needle, then placed my left hand at the base of the horse's neck to raise the jugular vein. Satisfied that I could clearly see where to place the needle, I said, 'Okay. Be prepared for him to jump.'

I had barely touched the needle tip to his fur when he sat back onto his haunches. As if he had been loaded into a cannon, he leapt forward, tearing out of Rodney's grasp. In the blink of an eye, the stallion was prancing against the fence, as far as he could get from us.

Rodney stood dumbfounded. He looked at me, wide-eyed. 'I didn't think he could move that quickly!'

I was not surprised. I might have been a child in Rodney's eyes, but I had dealt with hundreds of poorly handled horses and was very familiar with their reaction to the touch of a needle.

Rodney held up his left hand. A deep gash ran the circumference of most of the index finger. The blood trickled out, dripping off his knuckles as he held his palm upwards. His fingernail had been caught in the halter and torn off as the horse bolted.

I choked back some bile. I can cope with almost anything when it comes to animals. The idea of using a scalpel or suture on one of my own kind is another matter entirely, as is the sight of human blood.

'I'd better put a bandage on that,' I said.

I ran over to my car, reefed open the canopy to find the bandages and returned with a small wrap, which I wound firmly around Rodney's finger.

'It's just a scratch,' Rodney protested.

'It's almost ringbarked your finger. I'm taking you into the hospital.'

'I've never been to the doctor in my life,' he said, pulling himself up to full height.

That did it. If I didn't drive him into town, there was no way he was going to do it himself.

'Well, today's the day,' I said, and marched him towards my car.

I didn't want to frighten the man, so I didn't tell him I thought he'd lose the tip of his finger if it didn't get sutured back together immediately.

'Wait. I've got to make sure they've got water,' he said, gesturing his bandaged hand towards the horses.

I could see a hose and tap nearby.

'I'll do that. You sit down.'

I raced over to the tap and filled the buckets that sat within each pen. I left the gate for the bay's pen open, figuring that once he'd settled down, he would leave the main yard and find his water.

It was about a 20-minute drive to the nearest hospital in Menindee. Actually it's more of a clinic than a hospital, with a nurse on duty to administer first aid and refer anything more serious on to the Royal Flying Doctor Service. On the way in I called ahead to let them know we were coming.

'Rodney?' she exclaimed. 'It must be bad. He's never set foot in here in his life.'

Hearing that over the phone speaker, Rodney pointed out that the nurse had corroborated his own assertion that he was bulletproof, and repeated his doubts about the necessity of this trip. I continued driving. Along the way, Rodney proudly told me of all the other injuries and illnesses he'd survived in his lifetime while never needing to see a doctor. He was cut from the old cloth, where you only sought medical assistance if you were dying.

As we pulled into the clinic, the nurse was opening the front door to greet us. Perfect timing. Probably in her sixties, she had been the local nurse for many years and knew Rodney well.

'What have you done to yourself, you silly old man?' she said, fussing over him as she ushered us into the waiting room.

'Just bandage it up and I'll be right,' said Rodney.

'We'll see about that. I will be the one who decides what's going to happen.'

It was obvious Rodney was going to be looked after whether he wanted to be or not, so I excused myself. I had plenty of other clients booked in for the day. I heaved a sigh of relief as I returned to my car.

I called Rodney a week later.

'Thanks for taking me into the hospital,' he said. 'I would've lost my finger if you hadn't made me go. They're changing the bandage every two days and so far it looks like it will mend together. At one point they even wanted to fly me to Adelaide, but in the end they were able to patch me up in Broken Hill after I insisted there was no way I was going to the Big Smoke.'

I smiled at that. I felt for any medical professional who had to try and get Rodney to do as he was told. He was lucky he'd come across me and the nurse in Menindee.

As for his horses, they got to keep their knackers, as Rodney would so gracefully put it, for a bit longer. It was clear they were going to need to be calmer still before we tried the castrations again.

There was one other time when I've had to deal with a significant human injury – an injury of my own.

I was at home alone, Brendan out doing some work in a distant corner of the property. After rain the previous night, I figured it was a good chance to do some weeding in our garden. For a while it went well, but then the frayed hem of my jeans caught on some netting near a tree and I tripped over, driving my knee into a metal stake. Ouch. Once again I had managed to turn gardening into a dangerous sport. Blood oozed through my jeans. I swore, tore off the bottom of my already ripped shirt and wrapped the fabric tightly around the wound. Then I hobbled back to the house.

I sat down at the outside table and pulled off the makeshift bandage. I couldn't see much other than blood, so I undid my jeans and pulled them off, tossing them to the side as I assessed the degree of my wound. The cut was about five centimetres long, full-skin depth and about one centimetre into the fat pad underneath. I closed my eyes. This was going to need stitching, and as I was the only one around who knew how to do that, I was going to have to do some self-repair.

I sucked in a deep breath as I plucked up the courage to do what needed to be done. I went to the storage room where all my equipment is kept and grabbed a stitch-up kit that had been sent to me to try by one of the pharmaceutical companies (thanks guys!). The kit contained some pre-packaged sutures, gloves, local anaesthetic and antiseptic.

After returning to the living room, I made myself comfortable on the couch, straightening my leg and elevating it with cushions to give myself a good surgical view. I then cleansed the skin in preparation for surgery. But on the point of inserting the local anaesthetic, my bravery wavered. I could suture animals all day long, but was brought undone by the idea of sticking needles into a human, let alone this human. I couldn't do it. I sat the syringe of local on the surgical tray beside my instruments. How was I going to get this thing sutured? I couldn't justify taking myself 80 kilometres to the nearest hospital when it would take five seconds to do the job myself, but I couldn't bring myself to do it.

Then I was struck by an idea. Dad has had many surgeries done on himself. Perhaps he could inject the local for me?

Dad has a prosthetic leg. He'd elected to have it amputated below the knee after a lifetime of issues with his left foot. I was about ten at the time, James about eight, and I remember that when he came home from hospital, he was worried about how we children would react. After a brief moment of us looking at the stump with interest, James casually declared, 'It's a bit short!' Dad must have been holding his breath while waiting for our reaction, because he let out a relieved laugh. Ever since, though, he's had to frequently revisit his orthopaedic surgeon to have sebaceous cysts removed from the stump. I reasoned that with all his experiences in hospital, he should be an old hat with needles.

I rang the main house and he agreed to come to my assistance. He came in to find me perched up on the lounge. Unfazed, he pulled on the gloves that I'd readied for him. I passed him the syringe, after demonstrating how to insert the needle into my skin, then, just as he held the needle-tip to the edge of my wound, his hand started to shake. I realised this wasn't going to work.

'I thought you'd seen plenty of needles?' I said.

'I have. But I've never had to do the injecting,' he replied, wiping a bead of sweat from his brow.

What now? This was turning into a real circus. Maybe I should go into town after all.

'You'd better hand that back.' I held my hand open and he relinquished the syringe. 'Maybe you could pour a rum for us both?'

That idea drew an enthusiastic nod. This was a task he was practiced at!

He placed the glass of rum next to me on the coffee table, then said, 'I'll sit outside and have a smoke.'

'Good. That way you can still keep an eye on me and ensure I don't faint midway though surgery.' I was only half joking.

'Bloody hell! You're mad,' he said as he lit up a cigarette.

I took a large gulp of the rum, enough to burn my throat as I swallowed it. *Right, I can do this,* I thought. I inserted the needle and injected very slowly. It didn't hurt as much as I'd anticipated. I worked my way around the wound edge, injecting more anaesthetic to ensure the entire area was numb. *That wasn't too bad*, I reassured myself. But now for the real challenge.

I opened up the suture packet, picked up my needle drivers (scissor-like pliers for holding and working the needle) and grasped the pre-swaged (pre-threaded) needle. Okay. Deep breath. I went into surgeon mode, trying to dissociate my leg from myself. It crossed my mind mid-flight that human skin is not dissimilar to pig skin, and I was soon admiring a neat row of stitches as I wiped the wound clean and applied a firm bandage.

'Are you alright in there?' Dad enquired from his smoke-filled haze on the patio.

'Yep. All good,' I answered as I cleaned up my instruments.

I came outside with a fresh glass of rum for the two of us. Both our hands shook slightly as we sipped. *Next time I have an injury like that I'll go into town*, I thought.

SHORTCUT TO NOWHERE

I looked at the scratched-out map on the piece of paper in my hand.

'Just stick to the route and you can't miss it,' I'd been told.

Yeah, right. I'm always a prime candidate to stuff up even the clearest driving directions. Now I was undoubtedly lost. The landmarks around me were nothing like anything on my 'map'. I drove up and down an old fence line a dozen times, debating whether to continue left or right, with no confidence in either option.

I was on the first day of a road trip, but my diary contained enough calls in the immediate area around our place that I could plan to enjoy the luxury of returning home and sleeping in my own bed that night. I was up early to prepare for the two-hour drive to the first client, 180 kilometres away, all on dirt road. About 60 per cent of my driving is off the bitumen, though, bit by bit, new blacktop is being laid through the district.

As I threw my lunch pack into the car, I felt the cold, wet nose of a dog touch my leg, and looked down to see Bing, our scruffy little black Australian terrier. She looked up at me with pleading, impossible-to-resist eyes, her wagging tail adding weight to her case that she should be my assistant for the day. I bent down to pick her up, figuring she'd be good company for the drive. I placed her on the passenger seat, where she sniffed the upholstery before snuggling herself into a tight ball on the seat. I smiled at her peaceful, curled-up form as I reversed out of the garage.

I drove south-west from White Cliffs, through rocky hills interspersed with gibber flats. Gibbers are quartz pebbles, originally components of older conglomerate rocks, polished smooth by sand blown across the land for centuries. The landscape is littered with bluebush, a low-lying shrub with steel-blue coloured succulent leaves, and the occasional mulga tree. To the uneducated eye, it looks as barren as the moon, but this is sheep grazing country, traditionally good for wool growing as there is little to contaminate the fleece. In contrast, this country is too hard for the large hooves of cattle to bear.

Beth and Ken, whose station I was driving to, were wool producers with just a few cattle and goats. Like many of the people in this district, they had known me since I was in nappies. They'd asked me out to do various jobs on this visit, which was fairly typical. If you're going to get the vet to come all the way out to see you, you might as well get all your animals' needs attended to at once. I had a dozen working dogs and some household cats to vaccinate, a hundred rams to bleed before breeding season, and six horses needing dental exams.

Driving up to the entrance, there was no doubt I was at the right place. The name of the station was painted in large letters on a sign hanging over a closed four-metre-high gate. I swung the gate open, drove through, then closed and latched it behind me, obeying the golden rule in the bush: always leave a gate as you found it.

The driveway to the homestead wound around several rocky hills. I admired the view along the way, the still-early morning sun lending a pink hue to the hills. After seven kilometres, the corrugated iron roof of a house came into view. The house sat at the bottom of a hill with a creek below, a woolshed about half a kilometre further away on an open gibber flat. I could make out two utes parked over there, and a group of rams standing in the yards. I continued past the house with the hill to my right, then crossed the dry creek bed and drove up to the yards.

After pulling up, I wound down the windows so Bing would have some fresh air. It was a cool day and she would be safer staying in the car. She didn't even flutter an ear as I opened the door. What a life, I thought to myself with envy. I often joke that I work to keep my pets in the lifestyle to which they're accustomed, and Bing was proof of that in this moment.

Beth and Ken emerged from the vehicles, both dressed in jeans, elastic-sided boots, long-sleeved shirts and Akubra hats.

After saying our hellos, Ken suggested starting with the rams.

'Good idea. Where's the young bloke?' I said, referring to a farmhand they usually had around.

'We couldn't get the lad to help us today, but we have a Combi Clamp now,' she said, pointing to their sheep crush. It was the perfect setup for bleeding rams. A ramp led up to a raised platform, where each ram would be firmly held in place by moving side panels that closed when a person outside the crush stood on a plate along the outside. In the secured position, I could easily access the animal's neck from the front and their testicles from the other end.

'Looks perfect to me, Beth.' I smiled. 'I'll get you to be the scribe if you don't mind.'

Ken would catch each ram in the Combi Clamp and read out the identification number from its ear tag, which Beth would note in her neat handwriting. She would then hand me a labelled blood sampling tube.

I had two tasks to perform on each ram. The first was to find each animal's jugular vein and draw a blood sample from it. We test for a disease called ovine brucellosis, a sexually transmitted disease that affects the testicles, leading to infertility. These sheep had been shorn a few weeks before; the shorter wool made this job much easier because I could readily locate the jugular. The second task was to 'palpate' the testicles, which means checking, by feel, that they are normal and healthy, without any signs of disease.

The crush made the task quite easy, and we worked through the mob with relative ease, each of us performing our designated roles. After an hour we had completed the task and I had barely broken a sweat. The day was off to a flying start.

'This is the go,' I said, enthusiastically patting the side of their new crush.

'We've made allowances in our budget to upgrade our stock handling facilities over the past few years,' Ken said. 'It's getting harder to find workers, and this makes the work easier to do with just me and my scone burner.' He gave Beth a cheeky wink.

'We aren't getting any younger,' Beth said. 'The days of me wrangling sheep are long gone.'

'We'll have to get something like this when we can afford it,' I said. 'The first thing I did after moving home was replace our cattle crush, which was an accident waiting to happen.'

I told them how the old crush had been a museum piece. It had looked like a torture device sitting at the end of the race. It had a guillotine-style head catch, which required you to pull on a rope to open it and release the animal's head when you were done. But the rope often became rotten, breaking when you went to use it. The doors at the front of the crush were 'saloon' doors that swung forward, but without the release rope you had to lean underneath the neck of the beast to release the catch, then jump clear before the animal moved forward. It was so dangerous that Dad's livestock agent had been badgering him about it for years.

Ironically, that same agent played a role in Dad's buying a replacement. The agent had acted as auctioneer when a new cattle crush went up for auction at a local field day to raise money for charity. With more than a little coaxing and jeering about his ancient crush, Dad had been cajoled into making the winning bid. The next challenge was getting the thing installed. That auction took place three years before Brendan and I moved home, and it was still sitting on the red sand near the yard when we got there. Meanwhile, Dad kept using the old crush. Whenever I mentioned the need to replace it, the men always had more important jobs on their lists. More important, that is, until they saw me taking to the old crush with a cordless angle grinder one morning. All of a sudden they were all over it.

'If you need a man to do something, start the job yourself in a rough manner,' I said to Beth. 'They will soon race in to take over, for fear that the job won't be done to their standards.'

Beth laughed. 'The old saying is that if you want a job done properly, do it yourself. But failing that, if you can't do it properly, start the job in a haphazard manner with full enthusiasm. Those who can do it will come running.'

'You use the same tactic with mowing the lawn,' Ken said. 'Now, if we're done here I'll get my bike and take these fellas out to their paddock.'

'I've got the horses in the round yard next to the house,' Beth said.

After I invited her to join me for the drive over to the house, Beth opened the door to find my furry companion still snoozing blissfully.

'Bing, Bing,' I said, gently stroking her back to waken her.

Bing lazily opened an eye at me, then unfurled herself in a languid stretch. Seeing that she was in no hurry to make accommodations for our guest, I picked her up and placed her on my lap for the short drive.

'Climb aboard, Beth,' I said.

The round yard stood under some tall weeping gum trees. The horses paced around the yard, not used to being in such small confines. They were well-bred stock horses, brown or bay in colour. Beth was a campdrafter, meaning she took part in competitions involving working cattle on horseback. Think sheepdog trials, only with horses and cattle. She chose her horses carefully for this sport.

We climbed out of the car, leaving Bing to reclaim her former position on the seat. I opened the canopy and located the large silver case housing my equine dental equipment. I set about arranging my gear as Beth caught the first horse for me.

'I haven't had them seen to for a while,' Beth said. 'I try to get their teeth done whenever I have the chance, but with no vet around it hasn't been easy. Now that you're back in the district, I hope they'll be regularly attended to. This one's Rupert,' she added as she led a calm, bay gelding over to me.

I patted him gently down the neck and listened to his heart with my stethoscope.

'Give him a good scratch on the side of his eye,' I said. 'It will distract him as I slip the needle in.'

Rupert only twitched slightly as I injected his jugular vein. Within a few seconds his head drooped to the ground and his feet splayed as the sedation took full effect. I undid his halter, retying it loosely about his neck.

'He won't be going anywhere for a little while,' I said, then, noticing Beth's concern, I reassured her that these wobbles were perfectly normal. 'He won't fall. He's just relaxed and unstressed enough for me to work on his teeth.'

I inserted a heavy dental gag to keep the horse's mouth open and asked Beth to hold on to it while supporting the horse's head under his chin. Lifting the head to my eye height and looking down the long cavernous mouth, I could see ulcers along the outside edge of the tongue where the teeth had irritated the soft tissue. I inserted my hand and gave the mouth a thorough examination, which revealed a number of significant sharp points. These are common in horses that are hand fed. The teeth of a horse have exceptionally long roots and are always growing. If they spend most of their time out in pasture, they tend to naturally grind their teeth while masticating on grass. It's where this natural grinding is missing that intervention is often required.

'There's nothing to be concerned about here, but his teeth could definitely do with rasping to stop those mouth ulcers.'

I pulled out the PowerFloat, which is a battery-operated power tool I use specifically for this job. The tool uses a diamond-plated rotating disk that abrades the teeth without damaging soft tissue. In just a few minutes I had removed all the sharp points and given the mouth a satisfying final check. I released the gag, replaced the halter and allowed the horse's head to droop back down.

Beth stared at me in amazement. Without access to a vet, she'd only ever used lay-dentists to do the job. She couldn't believe how quickly and easily I had performed it.

'The last time I had someone do this job, they used a hand rasp. The horses hated it!'

The old hand rasp, which I used to use, is not only hard work but it also cuts through anything in its path, including your fingers.

Beth told me the dentists hadn't used sedation either, which would have been because they weren't qualified vets. Instead, Beth had to manually calm the horses by 'twitching', a method involving pinching the upper lip or an ear, which can help but is nowhere near as effective.

'Now I've seen them done like this, I won't have it any other way,' she said.

I worked through the other five horses reasonably quickly. All their teeth were in similar condition. By the end my forearms were aching – the downside of using a power tool that weighs about 20 kilograms.

We moved onto vaccinating the cats and dogs, which only took a little while, before Beth said, 'Smoko time. Coffee or tea?'

Coffee it was, always my first option. I was already beginning to sense that there was too much blood in my caffeine system. We sipped our drinks on the verandah, warmed by the sun. Ken soon joined us, kicking off his boots as he sat down, and we chatted idly over our cuppas.

After smoko, I looked at my watch and realised I'd better keep moving.

Standing up, I said, 'I have to go to the Johnston's. What's the best way from here?'

'There's a good shortcut,' said Ken. Travelling on the public roads, the trip was a 120-kilometre drive, but he assured me that I could shave 50 kilometres off using his 'unofficial' route. On a scrap piece of paper, Ken drew me a rough map and I listened intently as he described the way, taking note of the landmarks he mentioned.

'Just make sure you stay to the right at this fork,' he said, pointing at his map. 'Just stick to the route and you can't miss it.'

I did miss it.

Ken's words haunted me as I drove up and down the old barbed wire fence. Despite following Ken's map like a hawk, consulting it carefully as I came to every intersection and gate, the tracks I was driving on had been flooded a fortnight prior and there were no fresh tracks to guide me. I had obviously missed a washed-out track somewhere, only realising my mistake when I got to this fence line. I knew it was a boundary fence, but I was confused about which properties lay on either side. The names of two stations were on the gate, but the sign seemed to indicate that the next paddock was Beth and Ken's, whereas I thought I'd never left their place.

I looked over at Bing to see if she might share my anxiety, but she hadn't stirred and showed no sign of doing so. *Thanks for your help, Bing.*

Thinking I had better stay where I was, I tried to use the UHF radio to get some directions, but there was no answer. I was out of range. I swore loudly, causing Bing to raise her head from her nest as if to ask, 'Should I be worried here?'

'It's okay mate, we'll get out of here,' I said, not sure who I was trying to convince.

After chewing my lip with indecision, I eventually chose to drive along what appeared to be the slightly more well-maintained track. After a few kilometres, a relatively fresh set of tyre marks cut across the paddock and onto the road in front of me, so I decided to 'follow' that vehicle. As I drove it was soon clear that whoever I was following had been doing a water run. That meant I might be taking the long way, but it also meant I would eventually finish at someone's place. At least that was the theory. In practice I ended up going in a big circle and found myself back where I started, at the gate on the mysterious fence line.

For my next trick, I decided to go through the gate, even though my intuition told me that might return me to Beth and Ken. I continued to chastise myself for not turning around the moment I realised I was lost. A little way on I found another set of tyre marks, which I followed once again, and these eventually led me to a small house in the middle of a patch of thick scrub. I had no idea whose place I was on, but I was overjoyed to be somewhere.

I jumped out of the car and called out. No answer.

Walking up to the front door, it became clear that there was no one about. The house looked lived in – there were shoes by the door and dogs in the kennel by the shed – but whoever they were, they weren't here now. Damn. I didn't want to enter a stranger's house, and the lack of an antenna on the roof told me there wouldn't be a radio in there anyway. I dragged my feet back to the car, where Bing had sat up and was looking out the window as if to ask, 'Any luck?' I gave her head a quick scratch as I considered my next move.

It was only then that I noticed more tyre tracks. This time they followed a road alongside a powerline. Aha! The powerline had to lead to some form of civilisation. All powerlines lead to houses, towns or main roads, don't they?

Once again, my well-founded logic proved flawed. After following the powerline for a few kilometres, the tyre tracks darted off into the scrub. Who knows where they were going. I looked at the powerline again, then at the bush underneath it. Back when these lines were regularly serviced from the ground, all powerlines had graded roads underneath them. However, the wonders of modern technology and remote fault finding have replaced the need for these tracks to be maintained. In this case I could see that the road was still there, but with an encroaching growth of hopbush along it. Thankfully it was still only knee-high, so driveable in my ute.

Increasingly stressed, I continued down the powerline track, cringing every time I heard a bush scratch against the paintwork of my car. Had I not had Bing with me, I would have been a complete nervous wreck by now. At least with the scruffy little one curled up beside me, I didn't feel alone.

After about 10 kilometres of this, all the while wondering where on earth it would end and hoping like hell that I wasn't going to have to turn around and retrace my steps, I crossed a large sandy creek bed and finally came upon a homestead. As I emerged, I found Yvonne, one of our neighbours, walking along the road ahead of me.

'Christ! Ameliah! You scared the living daylights out of me,' she said as I pulled up alongside her.

'I'm bloody glad to have come across you!' I said.

Yvonne's son Brian emerged from the machinery shed. He looked at my car and then towards the creek, let out a low whistle and said, 'If you got through there, you got some driving skills, girl!'

I did my best to explain what had happened, knowing all along that everyone in the district was going to hear about this.

Finally I shrugged, deeply embarrassed with the whole situation. I sheepishly excused myself, and Bing and I set about finishing my rounds for the day, Bing having been unmoved through the whole affair. Needless to say, I avoided any potential shortcuts.

When I phoned Beth and Ken that night to tell them about how I'd managed to get lost, Ken had a brief chuckle before telling me that the gate was mislabelled. It had come off its hinges a few months previously, and in haste he had turned it over before refitting it. That had reversed the sign, which led to my confusion.

'I'd better do something about that for next time,' he said.

Thanks, but next time I'll be sticking to the main roads, I said to myself.

RAIN AND WEDDING VOWS

I was in the middle of one of my first road runs in early 2020 when it started to rain – enough rain to break the drought that had strangled much of New South Wales and Queensland for the past three years. Brendan and I had only been home for six months, but the outlook so far had been bleak. I kept my eye on rain radar images for building storm activity, not wanting to leave it too late to get home before the roads might be closed. I timed it well. The ute only just greased through the mud and arrived home before the wet set in properly, rain falling steadily over three days.

Before long, the previously parched ground couldn't hold any more moisture. The creek filled and water flowed its way into our lake.

Rainy days are the best for farmers. They're like forced holidays. There's nothing much we can do around the property, and even if we could, the chances of getting bogged are high. Better to ride it out and spend some quality time drinking coffee, occasionally checking the rain gauge and comparing our falls with those of neighbours. It does end up being an opportune time to catch up on office work, the sound and smell of rain reinvigorating our faith in being able to pay outstanding bills.

Times like this also prove that you are never really a grown up. Mud turns us all into children. Once the lake in front of our house began filling with water, Sue and I dug out the old inflatable swimming toys, including a particularly out of place, enormous plastic pink flamingo. Unfortunately, years in storage had not been kind to this bird, and after a couple of sessions of frolicking about on it, I had to put it down, so to speak. Eventually, as the lake's depth increased further, we even got to go waterskiing on the lake, something that only tends to happen every second or third summer even in non-drought periods.

The breaking of the drought gave me cause for optimism on a number of fronts.

In country like ours, the amount of feed in the paddocks, and therefore the number of cattle we can keep, is entirely dependent on how much rain we get. 'You make money out of mud,' or so they say. The extra feed provides the opportunity to 'stock up': to buy young animals and bring them to our place for fattening up. On top of that, breeding cattle are better fed and more likely to reproduce. The good season coincided with a period of high meat prices and low interest rates, so we really hit the trifecta.

Of course, we weren't the only farmers for whom things were looking up, and that would translate to more potential business for a young rural veterinarian working to establish her business.

It's amazing how quickly the mood shifts in the district. With signs of a good season, the atmosphere around the community becomes noticeably positive. Farmers regain their enthusiasm for their livelihood, purchasing livestock in large quantities to restock their lands. After drying out, dirt roads in the region are ground into powder as hundreds of trucks bring thousands of cattle into the district. With much of this country better suited to smaller-framed ruminants like sheep and goats in the long term, due to its semi-arid nature, good money can still be made by raising cattle in seasons when there's plenty of feed.

Finally, I had always planned to be married when our lake was full. No sooner had the creek started flowing through our neighbours' properties and towards the lake, than we were getting phone calls. 'Do I need to put on my suit and float down in my canoe to witness the wedding?' asked one caller.

The one downside of all this happening in 2020 was that it coincided with the COVID-19 pandemic. Being as remote as we are, we were less directly affected than many, especially those in the major cities. Nevertheless, as we started planning our wedding for October, we were forced to shift venues several times as the rules around gatherings constantly changed. We decided to stick to the date and let the chips fall where they may. If it was just us and the priest, so be it!

In the end it didn't come to that. We were married on a warm afternoon in spring, under the gum trees on the edge of the lake, the breeze off the water acting as nature's air conditioner to keep our small gathering cool. I rode in on horseback, sidesaddle, my lace train draped over my chestnut gelding's rump. Brendan looked like a tall glass of water in his three-piece silver-grey suit. Our celebrant, David Schrimpton, the local flying padre (yes, a flying man of the cloth), oversaw our 'I dos'. We all had a chuckle when he swallowed a fly mid-ceremony, pausing for a bout of retching before finishing the job of getting us hitched. We flew from the ceremony at home to White Cliffs, where we had our reception under the shed on the edge of the gymkhana racetrack, the place jazzed up with what seemed like five kilometres of fairy lights and some decorative gum leaves.

BLOATED BOVINES

The rain combined with warm autumn weather to cause green feed to sprout from the earth in abundance. It never fails to amaze me how quickly this country responds to moisture. Barren paddocks become lush fields of pasture within weeks. After years of dust storms, you would think that the seedbed would have been blown away, along with all the nutrient rich topsoil. Yet now there seemed to be an abundance of both.

The abundance of lush pasture does bring some health issues for animals, the main one being frothy bloat in cattle. Hungry cattle introduced to fresh pasture gorge themselves on the rich feed, which then churns into a frothy mass in their stomachs. Cattle regularly eradicate gasses from digestion by burping, but in this situation the froth blocks their ability to do so. Instead, the gas builds up, making the frothiness worse and causing them to blow up like a balloon. Frothy bloat isn't to be confused with gaseous bloat, which mainly occurs in animals being fed grain in feedlot situations. The two types of bloat have distinctly different methods of treatment.

One of the problems of not having a vet presence in our district for a long time was that old wives' tales and 'traditional' remedies to common conditions like bloat thrived.

On one occasion, I'd just returned to our house after being out in the paddock most of the day fixing flood gates, where the creek had washed down segments of fences. While thick leather gloves had protected my hands from barbed wire, my shirt sleeves bore many small tears and there were a few scratches on my arms. Done in, I was just about to plonk myself down in a comfy seat when my phone rang.

A panic-stricken voice came to me down the line. 'All our cows are going down!'

I proceeded to remove my boots and sweat-encrusted socks while the woman, who introduced herself as Marg, explained the situation.

'So let me get this straight,' I said when she'd finished. 'You found 20 dead cattle yesterday, you then gave them diesel and this morning another 15 are dead. So altogether there are now 35 dead out of a herd of 250?'

'Yes. What can we do?' Marg answered.

'You have a serious problem with frothy bloat,' I said.

I explained how frothy bloat occurs, then told her to stop giving them diesel as it wouldn't do them any good. That was probably what had killed the second lot of 15 overnight, not the bloat. The diesel Marg had given her cattle is an old-school remedy for bloat with exactly zero scientific basis. However, in desperation, people will try anything for their animals. When you find most of your cattle laid out dying in a grassy paddock, it incites sheer panic. And when there's no vet to contact, as there hadn't been in this district for years, you have to try something. You've heard, either from another farmer or a previous generation, that feeding them diesel can help, so you pour it into dishes and offer it to the cattle to drink. Cattle are inquisitive creatures, so they sniff the diesel and lap it up. Unfortunately, the highly toxic 'remedy' is readily absorbed into the bloodstream. You're left, as Marg was, with some cattle dying of frothy bloat and others dying of diesel poisoning.

'Can you come here?' Marg asked.

It was too late in the day to fly out to Marg's station, a two-hour flight away, and certainly too late to start the 500-kilometre drive by road.

'I can be there by eight tomorrow morning,' I said. 'How is your strip?'

The next morning, as the first rays of light beamed across the flat surface of our airstrip, I packed the various pieces of equipment and medications I would need. I was pleased with myself at being able to fit it all into the luggage compartment of my plane by leaning against the little flap door to lock it closed. After a walk-around check that nothing was amiss, I scurried over the wing and into the cockpit.

It was a windy day, the stiff northerly breeze providing plenty of lift as I took off into it. I was soon at my cruising altitude and heading eastwards, towards Bourke. The station I was going to claimed Louth as its nearest township, a tiny town of only around 50 people on the Darling River. It does have a maintained airstrip though, so if it turned out that I couldn't land on the station strip, I could divert to Louth, where Marg would fetch me in a vehicle.

As I flew eastwards, the land below became more and more green, masses of shimmering pasture waving about as the wind blew across it. Using landmarks on the ground, correlated with my chart and GPS, I made sure I stayed on course, and as I approached Louth I made a call on the VHF radio to let any other pilots know I was in the area. No one responded this time, but you never know who might be flying about.

I made another call 10 kilometres out from the station strip, announcing my intention to land there. Thankfully this strip was easy to find, the north-south aligned runway sitting in the middle of a flat, bare patch of ground with a powerline running parallel to it a safe distance away. After a flyover to inspect the surface from 200 feet above, I was satisfied that there was nothing there that could fold my wheels or snap the propeller. It did look like a tight fit though, a bit like a cricket pitch mown into a lush lawn. I lined up to land, and used full flaps then heavy pressure on the brakes to accommodate the short-field landing, skidding to a stop only metres from the end of the runway. Finally, I turned the plane to park her nose into the slight breeze on this cool autumn morning.

I stepped out onto the wing, enjoying the morning air as I waited for Marg to pick me up. Minutes later, a small buggy zoomed down from the opposite end of the strip, trailed by a pack of kelpies getting their morning exercise. As Marg pulled up alongside the plane, the four well-muscled dogs, two brown and two black-and-tan, jumped up into the back of the little vehicle.

'Good morning,' I said as I climbed down from the wing. 'Nice helpers you've got there.'

'Good of you to come,' she said. 'I haven't been out to the cattle yet this morning so I'm not sure what we'll find.'

Marg looked to be in her sixties, with curly silver hair. She was short and lean but had a farmer's firm handshake.

'I've brought everything we might need to deal with whatever we find,' I said with bravado.

Unpacking the luggage compartment, we loaded Marg's buggy with my examination box, medications inside, and my bloat bucket, which contained a funnel, a 40cm length of 7cm diameter poly pipe and two metres of clear stomach tubing. One of the dogs gave me a lick on the back of my neck as I settled into the passenger seat.

'Hey fella,' I said, stopping him from licking my face by giving him a firm pat on the head, keeping him at an arm's length.

'Rodge! You know better,' Marg berated him.

'It's okay, Marg. I've got an agreement going with him now.' I continued patting Rodge while we drove down the airstrip, over a cattle grid and along a track. I kept my other hand firmly around the exam box on my knee as Marg took a corner without any attempt to slow down. At a gate, I noticed thick clover beneath my feet. Marg drove along a fence before turning out into the paddock, following a creek.

'The ones I found yesterday were in along here,' Marg explained as the buggy pushed through tall grass.

'It doesn't surprise me that they got bloat off this,' I said, waving my arm at the feed.

'Yes. I didn't think when I put them into this paddock. When I brought them from Dubbo two months ago, they were on my higher country. After the creek dried up I thought they could clean it up. I didn't think the feed would be too rich. But since I put them in here, they've been like kids let loose in a lolly shop.'

The buggy pushed past a thick clump of trees into an open floodplain where the herd of cattle was grazing, spread out at random. As we approached, I could see that several were sitting, slow to rise, their abdomens swollen with grass. After Marg came to a halt in the middle of the floodplain, it was clear that these cattle had been stuffing themselves. They were borderline obese, fat wobbling about their chunky brown frames as they walked and grazed. Marg had told me there should be 250 in the paddock. On a quick count, I estimated 20 per cent of them were showing obvious signs of bloat.

'As a starting point, we need to get them out of here,' I said. 'If they stay in this paddock, you will only lose more cattle. I'll treat those that can't walk as we come across them.'

Marg frowned, looked out at the herd, considering my advice. She nodded. 'I'll give Ben, my manager, a call. He shouldn't be far away.'

Marg called Ben over the two-way radio and explained the plan.

'I'm coming through Deadman's Paddock, I'll open the gate for the cattle,' he said.

'Thanks Ben. I'll start pushing them up there. If you could come to the floodplain, most of them are here.'

We slowly started mustering the cattle towards the northern side of the paddock, where the gate Ben had opened into a less rich paddock was located. Ben, a man of about my age, soon joined us on a motorbike. I was grateful to have the help, as there appeared to be a fair bit of work to do. There were at least a dozen large cows who could not get to their feet.

I asked Marg to drive the buggy over to where three cows were sitting close together. I then pulled out the tubing and piece of poly pipe. My bovine audience gave me a quizzical look.

'I need to put a tube down their throats. I'll administer fluids and bloat oil that will settle the froth, and then they'll be able to start burping off the gas as they normally would. I'll place the poly pipe in their mouth so that when they chew, they won't chomp on the tubing.' Bloat oil is a mineral oil blend created specifically for this purpose – very different from diesel fuel.

Ben pointed at the piece of poly. 'So this protects the tubing?'

'Exactly,' I said.

Marg and Ben helped me by passing pieces of equipment as I needed them. I stood at the right shoulder of the first cow, lifting the cow's head by placing my hand over her jaw into the upper corner of the mouth, then turning her head towards me. I inserted the poly pipe so that it was all the way at the back of her mouth, then fed the tubing through the pipe to the back of her throat. When I felt her swallowing, I pushed the tube down into her oesophagus, seeing the flutter of the end of the tube pass down the left side of her neck. As it entered the stomach, the end of the tube made a gurgling noise and I copped the whiff of grassy gas up my nose. Satisfied that I had successfully placed the end of the tube into the stomach, I attached the funnel to the outside end of the tubing, into which I asked Ben to pour 20 litres of water, followed by a few litres of bloat oil.

He picked up the tub of water, and as he began pouring it into the funnel, I leaned on the shoulder of the cow, cradling her head in my left arm while holding the funnel upwards with my right. As the liquid ran down the tubing, the cow chewed on the poly pipe, making the grunting noises that are music to the ears of a vet. They are the cow's way of saying thanks, grateful grunts as they are rehydrated. Once the last of the liquids disappeared down the tubing, I kinked off the tube and pulled it straight out, then removed the poly pipe from her mouth as well. I stepped back as the cow swung her head free. She already appeared much brighter. She looked about and, with a bit of effort, managed to roll onto her feet, standing for a few seconds as if regaining composure after such an undignified ordeal, then walked off to join the main herd that was still making its way towards the next paddock.

Ben and Marg exchanged impressed nods before looking back to me.

'Do you need to be a vet to do that?' Marg asked.

'No. If you're happy to have a go, I'll get each of you to tube the next few cows.'

I took their eager nods as agreement, and on the next cow Marg attempted to tube the animal. After a few tries at grabbing the mouth, she eventually got the correct grasp over the head and was able to complete the rest of the process. After administering the fluids, this cow also looked much brighter, but she was still unable to stand.

'Don't be discouraged,' I said. 'Sometimes they need several days of nursing care before they stand up. Sometimes they can't get up at all, despite being lifted. That's a risk with these bigger cows. They're so heavy that when they lie down for a long time, they can't feel their legs anymore because the blood flow to them is restricted. It's similar to when we get pins and needles from sitting down for too long.'

Marg gave the cow a thoughtful gaze. 'So we should be lifting them up?'

'Yes. Ideally lift them up two or three times a day for 15 minutes at a time. Then lay them down on the opposite side you found them to encourage blood flow.'

Ben looked doubtful.

'Yes, nursing large animals is a lot of work. But it will make the difference between life and death in this situation,' I said.

He mulled this over and then asked, 'At what point do you give up?'

'I had a patient that was down for a month once. She was a dairy cow that had bad post-calving paralysis. After a month of the farmer nursing her, bedding her down in the hay shed on thick straw, she eventually managed to stand up. That is the longest I have known a farmer to persist in nursing a down cow. My approach is that if they don't make a considerable improvement within a week of being regularly lifted, that's when I would consider pulling the pin. But of course it's up to you and what you can do to assist in easing her suffering. If you can't offer that kind of supportive care, there is no point prolonging the inevitable.'

They seemed appreciative of this real-world advice. I'm not a vet who thinks less of people who don't move heaven and earth to do everything for an animal. You can only do what you're able to, and that differs for everybody. Better an animal is put down than forced to live in suffering.

We continued tubing the rest of the down cows, taking turns at inserting the tube. Many of the cows stood up afterwards with some extra encouragement. It was almost midday by the time we had finished the job, by which time both Marg and Ben had become expert tubers.

Marg looked about the paddock as we finished tubing the last cow. 'Well I think we've earned our lunch today, Ben. Will you join us?' she said to me.

Turned out the cows weren't the only beings whose stomachs had been rumbling. 'I'd love to,' I said, trying to keep it casual and not appear like a ravenous street urchin.

Ben held up the tubing. 'This is quite effective! I'll admit I had my doubts when I watched you do the first cow, but now I can see the value in treating them.'

'It doesn't cost much to do,' I said with a smile. 'You only need oil, water and the plastic gear.' Turning to Marg I added, 'And you won't need to pay me to come out here every time now that you can do it yourselves.'

On the verandah of Marg's house, we shared a plate of sandwiches, the plate placed in the middle of the table as an open invitation to help ourselves. Only the fact that I'd been brought up with some manners prevented me from devouring them all. Marg poured freshly brewed coffee into a dainty china cup for me. It was the good china, with its delicate floral pattern and gold rim, reserved in most farmhouses for special guests. I felt very honoured.

As I made to leave, Marg couldn't express her appreciation enough. She kept shaking my hand with both of hers, saying, 'You have just saved me thousands of dollars. I only wish I'd rung you earlier, before putting the diesel out.'

I patted her arm. 'I understand you were looking for an easy remedy. It's the natural thing to do. But moving them off the rich pasture before it's too late is the easiest remedy, the next being the tubing.'

I went on to explain that to prevent bloat in the first place, the cattle need to be introduced to such pasture gradually, and shouldn't be given the chance to gorge on it. I also mentioned that the bloat blocks, or licks, you can buy at the co-ops are actually manufactured for grain bloat, rather than frothy bloat, so they wouldn't really be a viable solution in Marg's circumstances.

Marg and Ben both took this information on board. Marg asked Ben if he could drive the tractor out that afternoon and start lifting the immobile cows. With that he excused himself. I helped Marg load the dishwasher before she took me back to my plane.

'Thank you again!' she said, waving as I fired up the engine.

As I took off, I looked down and could see the tractor ambling along the creek towards the cows that had remained down. I could see that several of them were already standing on their own. There is nothing more satisfying than seeing an animal make a complete turnaround; from being on the brink of death to back on their feet in a matter of minutes.

Marg rang me a week later with an update. Two of the down cows had to be put down, but the other 18 had made a full recovery with nursing care.

BLEEDING THE RAMS

The air was as smooth as fine chocolate. Not a single bump of turbulence. I had taken off at dawn, as the first hints of light appeared on the horizon. Watching the sunrise from the cockpit gives me the sensation that I could be the queen of the land, a bit like the opening scene of *The Lion King* when the first rays of light hit the top of Pride Rock. I hummed tunes happily to myself as I sailed along. This is what my life was made for.

I was heading south, a northerly tail wind giving me good speed. My groundspeed was 145 knots, which equates to about 270 kilometres per hour. It's a rare blessing to have a tail wind when you are embarking upon a long flight. In this case it took me just two hours to get to the sheep station I was heading to; near Balranald, not far from the Victorian border. As I peered down through the cockpit window, the landscape below was a vast spread of red, with green tinges where grass was beginning to sprout after rain just a week earlier.

The Ghawns had a large merino flock, wool production being their main enterprise, and I had been asked to examine their rams with blood samples and palpitation of the testicles, just as I had done earlier for Beth and Ken's herd.

I'd been honest when asked about bleeding the rams. 'I can do it, although many people use the government vet as they are half the cost of me,' I explained to Mr Ghawn.

He was unperturbed by this information. 'I'd like you to come. We've used the DPI before but I'd rather someone with practical knowledge.'

Flattered by that, I agreed to fly down. There were 300 of them, a considerable number. Not many people had managed to get through the drought with many sheep, so I was a little intimidated when Mr Ghawn casually mentioned that they had 'about 20,000' ewes. Brendan and I were proud of the mob of 500 Dorper/Aussie White–cross sheep that we'd bought recently and were raising for meat, but the Ghawns' numbers made us look like hobby farmers.

I estimated that getting through all these rams would take me a full morning, likely four hours, five if it included smoko. Usually as a visitor you're asked to join in for a cuppa, though that custom is slowly fading away as farms become corporatised. Either way, with the two-hour flight down and three hours back into the wind, the job was going to take me a full day.

I watched the GPS closely as I came closer to the Ghawns' station. The land down their way was much greener, practically iridescent, after being inundated with rain a few weeks earlier. According to the coordinates I'd been given, the airstrip should have been on my nose, but it was hard to see anything other than green pastures. I was pretty good at picking out red runway in red surroundings, but less practiced at telling green from green. I pulled back power to descend lower, and a few white dots came into focus: the painted tyres marking the runway were only just visible through the high grass. Nevertheless, as I did my low pass to check the strip, I could see the runway itself had been mowed short.

I turned my bird around so as to land into the northerly wind, checking all my instruments and slowing the plane down. Landing into the wind is always a pilot's preferred option. The wind holds the aircraft up a little, which helps slow it down for a gentle touchdown. If you can't land directly into the wind – the orientation of a runway obviously can't be changed – you'll choose to land as close to into the wind as possible. Occasionally the wind will be perpendicular to the runway, which can be challenging and even dangerous if it's strong enough.

On my final approach I could make out a station car driving towards the strip from a nearby homestead. My wheels met the grass strip ever-so-smoothly and I allowed myself a mental fist pump as I braked.

As I shut down the engine and clambered onto the wing, the car pulled up alongside.

'G'day, Mr Ghawn. Your country is looking beautiful. I'm not used to finding green strips,' I said.

Mr Ghawn stood about six feet (183cm) tall, sandy hair underneath a floppy Akubra. He was dressed ready for the day's work, in jeans and a long-sleeved khaki work shirt.

As he shook my hand, he commented on my nice landing. Turned out he was a pilot too.

The breeze was only light, but as I was going to be there all day, and the wind would likely pick up, I tied the plane down anyway. I then retrieved the equipment I would need, which wasn't much for this task: needles, blood tubes, paper and gloves. I placed my bag in the back of the ute, climbed into the passenger seat, and enjoyed the lush scenery as Mr Ghawn drove me to the sheep yards.

Standing in the yards were 300 of the biggest merino rams I have ever seen, a mix of polled (hornless) and horned. They were due to be shorn in a month or so, after which they would be joined with the ewes. I hoped those lady sheep had the strong legs they'd need to hold up underneath these mammoths. The long wool told me I was in for a lengthy morning, as finding the jugular vein to take a blood sample is always harder through a woolly jumper.

Mr Ghawn had organised to have two workers help us out for the day. They arrived with a pack of fit-looking, shiny-coated kelpies, the whole team in an old Suzuki four-wheel-drive ute that drove in behind us as we parked. This was going to be a more traditional process than the modern one Ken and Beth had introduced me to with their Combi Clamp.

'G'day, I'm Jess,' said the drop-dead-gorgeous blonde girl who strode from the driver's seat to shake my hand.

'Ameliah,' I replied, only a little awed by this confident woman.

A thin young man emerged from behind the ute.

'I'm Lance,' he said, proffering his hand. He was the same height as me, Jess clearly the tallest and most imposing of us.

Jess and Lance jumped the rails of the yard and got to work pushing the rams into the narrow drenching race. I sorted through my sampling equipment, organising it neatly on the fold-out table beside the race, then showed Mr Ghawn how to label the tubes and correctly write the identification of each ram onto the form.

Once the first lot of rams was in the race, the hard work began. Jess was the main muscle, holding the head of each ram steady as I collected a blood sample from the neck. Lance held their rears, ensuring they couldn't move backwards. After taking the sample, I palpated the testicles of each ram, calling out any issues I discovered for Mr Ghawn to note on the form. We had to take some care when dealing with the horned rams, who knew how to inflict pain by ramming their heads up against the side of the race.

The first batch always took the longest to do on these jobs. It takes the initial run to get into the rhythm of catching the head and taking blood from the neck, while simultaneously calling out the identification tag number to the scribe, then seamlessly moving to the rear of the animal to feel the testicles.

'Ram ID number 214, sample number 38,' I'd call out as Jess and Lance wrangled the 38th ram in the queue.

We were keeping Mr Ghawn busy as he wrote frantically and readied the next test tube for me. He'd pass me the needle and the tube, and I would lean over the rail of the yard and insert the needle into the side of the neck where the jugular vein should be. Sometimes it took some repositioning to find the right spot amongst the thick folds of wool.

At one point Lance let out a sudden cry of pain after an impatient ram head-butted him in the most sensitive area of his nether regions.

I put my hand on his shoulder to steady him as he doubled over.

'Maybe you should swap places with Jess for a while,' I suggested.

He nodded, unable to speak. Jess swapped roles with him, taking hold of the rams' back ends while he took charge of the heads.

We finished the first run of 50 rams in under an hour, and after that each run got faster as we got into the rhythm. As we started working at a comfortable pace, we were able to chat about all manner of topics. The task of palpating rams lends itself to humorous banter.

'How would mine stack up?,' said Lance at one point, wiggling his bum next to a ram as I felt around the woolly scrotum.

'If you're game I'll give you an examination, although your voice may remain a few octaves higher for quite a while afterwards,' I said with a laugh.

'Yeah, I been watchin' you with these fellas. I reckon I'll keep my dangle berries tucked up,' Lance said.

'Yours wouldn't be big enough to feel anyway,' added Jess.

'We all know you've got the biggest balls here, Jess,' said Lance.

Jess shrugged and we all had a chuckle. He was probably right. Jess was clearly a capable woman, quite forthright even with Mr Ghawn, her employer. He was easygoing though, and didn't take offence. He appreciated having someone with initiative around.

I was interested to know whether this hardworking lass had found a local bloke to keep her in the area. I got straight to the point.

'Have you got a fella?'

Mr Ghawn snorted before Jess could reply. 'She's a hard marker, our Jess here.'

'Nothing wrong with having high standards. But there surely must be a few single, local blokes who might be alright?' I asked Jess.

'Nah, they've all got baggage. Seems I've missed the boat. All the blokes are either married by the time they're in their thirties, or if they're not, it's for a good reason.'

I nodded. 'I had to go 800 kays away from home to find someone. But I do know of a few boys up our way who are single.'

I listed off the names that came to my mind. Jess had either met or knew of each of them, and responded with a reason why they weren't potential love interests.

I gave up, turning to Mr Ghawn. 'You're right, she's a hard marker.'

He laughed. 'I tried to tell you. Jess is too hard on them.'

'I don't know what you mean,' said Jess as she and Lance wrestled another ram into submission. 'All I want is someone who doesn't smoke, has a bit of go about them and isn't a wanker.'

'Maybe you should take the advice that I was given: marry rich and learn to love them later!' I cheekily suggested.

'How's that workin' for ya?' Jess asked as I took another blood sample.

I chewed my lip in concentration on my task before I replied.

'Well, Brendan and I both said we were going to marry wealthy. But it turns out that rubbing two cents together doesn't equal a dollar.'

That got a laugh out of everyone. In the end we all agreed that finding someone who didn't come with baggage narrowed the options.

'I'd like to see Jess settled with a local fella, or someone who wants to make a life out here,' said Mr Ghawn. 'We don't want her to leave. She's a great help to have.'

Mr Ghawn was another farmer who had found it difficult to hire employees due to the challenge of attracting and keeping young people in the bush. He understood that when someone young, such as Jess, moves into a community without any ties to it, the community needs to do what they can to try and keep them in the area. Hopefully that would eventually mean she found a partner in life, as running a property is a lonely life on your own. In the meantime, Mr Ghawn's strategy for keeping Jess around was to offer her a long-term lease on some of his land, on which she could run her own flock of sheep.

'I have my own dowry sorted,' joked Jess. 'I come with ten handy working dogs, three horses, a motorbike, a car, a horse float and a mob of fine-wool merinos.'

'Seems to me you've got everything you need,' I said.

'I *would* like a nice fella,' she said with a more serious note.

'I'll put an ad up for you,' I said.

'Seriously?' She raised an eyebrow at me.

'Yeah. It'll say, "Wanted: man with big chequebook, penis to match",' I said with a wink.

At that Mr Ghawn fell over in laughter, and the shock on Jess's face melted as she too doubled over. It took a few minutes to regain our composure before we continued with the job at hand, occasional fits of giggles continuing for a little while.

Since that first visit, Jess and I have got to know each other a bit and we get along well, the two of us young women determined to do our own thing, with or without a significant other. Though of course, should any nice, good-looking fella, free of baggage and keen on life in the country, read this and want to get in touch with her ...

MY OLD MATE

Old Mr Love lived on his own in a small weatherboard and corrugated-iron-roofed house on 'the mission', the name commonly given to a government housing cul-de-sac on the outskirts of a town. His house was like those of all his neighbours who, like him, are First Nations Australians and some of the poorest members of our society.

In his semi-retirement, Mr Love spent most of his days tinkering on old machinery, fixing up bits and pieces for others in return for his 'sugar and tobacco' (an old term for wages). His yard housed a random assortment of old tractors and motors, all placed in neat rows, the grass and weeds around them kept short. He didn't have much but didn't want for much either. He just needed something to do and someone to care for. Since his wife had died, the someone he was caring for was an aging blue heeler with the not-so-imaginative name of Red.

I'd visited Mr Love a few times over the years. Like many in this community, he didn't have a phone, so if he needed to see me he would wander into the local council offices and ask someone in there to call me. Even some who had a phone of their own would do this because, for whatever reason, they found having to call me intimidating.

When I called in on Mr Love, there was always a cup of tea on offer and I could never say no, even though I prefer coffee. He was from a time when coffee was instant and undrinkably bitter, so tea was all he drank. While these visits were usually premised on Red needing a worming tablet or a check-up for some minor ailment, I knew they were often really about Mr Love wanting a chat with someone who had an interest in his stories. Over our tea, I would hear the tales of the past. He sat across from me, his hair white and kept neatly short like his lawn. Creases in the corners of his eyes hinted at his kind nature, while callouses on his hands and grease embedded in his knuckles were reminders of a lifetime of hard work.

Back in the day, Mr Love had been a stockman, a real old-fashioned drover, who worked with local landowners including my grandfather, Bill. With his team, he would ride his horse and drive stock along the side of the road during dry periods. If they came across water, they'd pause for the stock to take a drink. Mr Love and his mates would fill a billy from a canvas water bag, boil the water, and add tea leaves from a tuckerbag. Afterwards they'd take a short nap on their saddle blankets before re-mounting and moving the mob onwards. This sort of droving is pretty much a thing of the past now, at least in western New South Wales. When it is done, the herding work is conducted on motorbikes rather than horses. I enjoyed hearing these stories of simpler times.

Visiting the mission was confronting on occasion. The place has a stigma, which unfortunately exemplifies the inequality caused by two hundred years of European oppression of First Nations people. Some houses are missing doors and floorboards, the timber being needed for firewood. Often an old blanket hangs across the front doorway. Small sedan cars are parked out on the footpath with windows smashed and wheels missing. I'm told crime rates are high.

All of this is representative of a vicious cycle of poverty in which generations have been disenfranchised and left almost completely dependent on welfare. When the only way to break out of the cycle is to leave the families they treasure and seek opportunities elsewhere, I can understand why many prefer not to do so.

I've been able to get to know others in the community like Mr Love, who treasure their animals enough to contact me, despite how intimidating some find it. Usually in my job, anyone who calls me 'Doctor' is doing it with cheek or offensive humour, but with those I visit on the mission, I'm addressed as 'Doctor' or 'Missus Vet' with genuine respect. I once tried to get Mr Love to call me Ameliah. His response was, 'No, Missus Vet. You call me properly, I call you properly.' Fair enough.

*

One day I was driving past Mr Love's place when he waved me in.

'Something's really not right with Red,' he said.

I looked over to the patio where Red always slept on a threadbare couch. From a distance he looked to be dozing peacefully.

'He always comes for a wander around the yard in the morning,' said Mr Love, 'but lately all he does is lie on that sofa.'

I hopped out of the ute and collected my exam bag from the back, then followed Mr Love onto the patio. When I knelt in front of the couch, Red stirred a little and gave us a small wag of his tail in acknowledgement of our presence. Mr Love sat beside his mate and stroked his back, while I proceeded to examine the dog.

His heart was beating unusually quickly and his pulse felt weak.

'I suspect he's having some issues with his ticker. If you like I can do some X-rays on his chest to get a better idea of what's going on?'

Mr Love looked up. 'You got an X-ray machine with you?'

'Yep. It's a portable one, designed for horses, but it will take the shots we need of Red's heart.'

With some help, I retrieved the various boxes that housed the X-ray generator, laptop and processor, and had the system set up in about 15 minutes.

Red lay obediently on top of a digital X-ray plate as we donned heavy lead gowns. I lifted the 20-kilogram generator and held it over the dog, steadying my arms as much as I possibly could while holding the weighty rectangular box at a precarious angle away from my body.

'X-ray,' I called as I clicked the button to take an image. I sat the generator down and turned it off to prevent any inadvertent exposure while I checked the picture. Mr Love was about to remove his gown, but I placed my hand over the sash to stop him. It's hard work getting an animal patient to lie still for a single X-ray, and there's a real knack to snapping the image while the patient is perfectly still. That only gets harder every time you have to re-do it. So, the vets' rule for taking X-rays is to keep your lead gown on until all images have been processed. This seems to appease the vet gods, so that you don't have to re-dress and take more images because the first ones are blurry.

When a clear, sharp image of Red's chest appeared on the laptop screen I let out a breath of relief. The picture showed up all the relevant anatomy in perfect clarity.

'Righto, now you can take off the gown,' I said cheerfully.

Pointing to Red's heart on the photo, I explained the situation to Mr Love. 'He has left-sided heart failure, likely due to a leaky valve within the left ventricle. His heart is enlarged as it's been working hard to compensate. The good news is that there are meds we can put him on to make the heart work more effectively and avoid a collapse.'

Unfortunately one of those drugs was expensive, about $200 a month for a 30-kilogram dog like Red. Numbers like this can come as a shock to our clients. We're very lucky in Australia to have a medical system for humans that makes most drugs much cheaper than their real cost, but as there is no Medicare for pets, we have to dispense veterinary medications, which are no less costly than human ones, at full price.

Luckily this time I had some out-of-date, but perfectly safe, donated medication I was able to offer Mr Love in the short term.

'I won't always have a supply of this to offer you, but when I receive any I'll make sure I put it aside for you,' I said.

Mr Love was grateful. 'I understand. I'll just have to find an extra motor to fix each month, and that will pay for them. I've got a bit of work lined up so it won't be a problem paying for his meds.' He waved his hand towards the line up of old vehicles parked in the yard.

Red survived another six months, but medications can only do so much. He eventually became quite lethargic and passed away peacefully in his sleep. Mr Love buried him in his yard, placing a stone he had carved into the shape of a dog atop the mound.

TIBOOBURRA COCKY

Driving a couple of hundred kilometres past Mr Love's place brings me to Tibooburra, the most north-western township in New South Wales. It's tucked up in the top-left corner of the state, 1187 kilometres from Sydney. It is a well-known tourist stop for grey nomads and other outback adventurers; the last chance to resupply before they head into miles of uninhabitable desert country on their way to Sturt National Park or even more remote places like Innamincka in South Australia.

Tibooburra only has a population of a hundred or so, but it is also home to one of the most infamous pet birds that has ever existed. Barney the cockatoo lives at TJ's Roadhouse, though he is named after the old publican of the Family Hotel. Unlike his namesake, the bird is not a polite, mild-mannered citizen. A sign above his portable cage reads: 'DO NOT INSERT FINGERS. WILL BITE'.

Despite the warning, many a larrikin has played finger roulette with Barney, mostly young blokes who see Barney as the perfect test of their manhood. They soon find out that Barney holds nothing back. Once he latches onto a fleshy digit, he applies a vice-like clamp with his beak. Inevitably, blood is drawn as the brave (stupid) instigator of the game yanks their finger back. The cockatoo then stands proudly on his perch as if to say, 'I told you so, dickhead.' I'm pretty sure that if he were human, profanity would be liberally peppered throughout his speech. All of this is a great source of entertainment for locals and tourists, who watch the goings-on from the tables next to the window in the servo restaurant.

Jacko and his wife, Mavis, have run the roadhouse for many years. Actually, it's really Mavis who does the running. All the businesses in Tibooburra are owned and operated by women, making this far-flung outback town one of the most socially progressive communities in Australia.

Mavis is a slim woman in her seventies, with short-cropped white hair, while Jacko has the build typical of many men in semi-retirement. As he himself says, he decided carrying a six-pack in front was overrated, so he carries a keg instead. Almost always wearing a shirt, shorts and sandals, Jacko entertains tourists with his tall tales about bush life, while Mavis puts their food and coffee orders through the till.

On my monthly road runs, I have come to know most of the servos along the way. I try to support them all by buying fuel, food or both. What goes around comes around in the bush's circular economy, and it helps to keep these small businesses going, especially in times when there aren't many tourists passing through.

On my last visit though town, Jack mentioned that Barney could do with a good check-over. He was concerned about a lump under the bird's eye. I agreed that I would have a look on my next trip, before which I would arm myself with an arsenal of restraints along with my gaseous anaesthetic machine. Most wildlife and birds are anaesthetised with gas in order to safely examine them, with the benefit that it also leads to less distress on the animal's part.

I met Jacko at the back of the shop, where we agreed it would be best if he wheeled the pesky bird away from the prying eyes of the public. While my task was bound to be entertaining, it may also have been stressful for Barney, not to mention his vet, to have an audience. Mavis had thoughtfully placed a pile of old towels in the back room, where there were also towers of empty cardboard boxes and a line of spare freezers along the wall. I checked that the room's two doors were able to close properly, which minimised the chances of escape should Barney get away from me. Birds have an innate ability to find escape routes.

I'd parked near the back door as my anaesthetic machine is heavy and awkward. I also had to hoist out my oxygen generator, a rectangular box standing 80cm tall and weighing 25 kilograms. Moving it was like carting a small bear. With this equipment and a few other bits and pieces wrestled into the back room, it was time to do battle with Barney.

I opened the rear door into the shop to find Jacko manoeuvring Barney's cage past display shelves towards me. Barney was making a few squawks of protest, so I grabbed one of Mavis's towels and threw it over the cage. Reducing the light normally helps to calm stressed animals, though in this case it did not work. Rather, Barney seemed to turn up his volume as we approached the storage room.

We propped the door ajar, easing the cage through the snug doorway. By the time we'd done that, we already had sweat running down our faces. I wiped my forehead with the back of my shirt sleeve and closed the door firmly, locking the two of us, and Barney, into the room. Thankfully the windows had flyscreens, so we were able to open two large double bay windows on either side of the back door. Not only was the fresh air a welcome relief, but it would prevent us from becoming dizzy should any anaesthetic gas escape.

I pulled out my anaesthetic machine, connected it to the oxygen generator and checked for leaks in the system, then attached a large cone-shaped mask to the end of the gas line. The system would administer a blend of sedative gas and oxygen, and my plan was to put the mask over Barney's head and hold it there for a few breaths until he was calm enough to handle. I removed the towel from the cage, ready for action.

Barney sat on the uppermost perch, at my eye level. Up close I could admire his crisp white feathers and the streaks of bright yellow in his comb and under the wings. He had a grey beak and grey ring of skin about his eyes, and below his left eye was the pea-sized lump Jacko had been concerned about. He was not impressed at this looking over. In fact, if a bird could wear a murderous expression, this was it. I took a deep breath. If Barney was prepared to seek vengeance for the disruption to his routine, I needed to be ready for war.

'I've got an old tin he likes to play with,' said Jacko. 'He often puts it on his head, like Ned Kelly. Maybe I could see if he'll voluntarily put his head inside it?'

'Go for it,' I said. 'If he puts his head into the tin, I might be able to wrap a towel around him, and get him out of the cage with all my fingers intact.'

Jacko went into the shop and returned with the steel can. I thought it would be perfect. He wouldn't be able to bite through it, and he shouldn't feel stressed if he played with it as a game. Jacko opened the cage and gingerly presented the tin, open end upwards, towards Barney. Barney looked down at the tin for a moment, then looked at me, then back at Jacko. Quick as a flash, he snatched the open end of the can with his beak and took it off Jacko. He toyed with it for several minutes, gnawing around the open rim of the can while clasping the bottom with his claws. I was impressed by his dexterity, by how his comparatively small feet were able to grasp the edge of the tin quite firmly. Jacko and I held our breath. Barney continued to play, then after a few more seemingly playful screeches, he tipped his head down and tossed the tin onto his head using his foot.

At that moment, Jacko opened the cage door and I threw a towel over the bird's wings, but as I tried to wrap my hands around him he let out a mighty shriek and shook the tin from his head, then chomped down into the towel, only narrowly missing my fingers. I whipped my arms out of the cage, letting the towel fall to the bottom as Barney shrugged it off.

The very cross cocky growled at us like a dog, shuffling towards us on his perch and giving us the dirtiest stink-eye possible. I threw another towel from the pile over the cage and took a step back.

Time for Plan B.

Trying the tin-can plan again would only stress Barney further, leading to injury either to him or, more likely, to one of us.

'Towels aren't going to cut it,' I said to Jack. 'Do you have any welding gloves?'

While he left the room to have a look, I sat quietly, giving both myself and Barney a few minutes to calm down. Under the towel over the cage, I could hear Barney pacing up and down his perch like a prison inmate plotting his escape.

Mavis returned, proffering a pair of thick, black, elbow-length welding gloves. 'Will these do?'

I accepted them gratefully and pulled them on. If these didn't work, nothing else was going to. As Jacko arrived back in the room, I could hear the chorus of tourists chattering out the front before he closed the door again. *Great,* I thought. *They might not see the drama unfolding in here, but they'll definitely hear it!*

'It's going to take two of us to get him,' I said. 'I'll try to wrap him in the towel again, and you put that tin over his head and hold it in place while I draw him out of the cage.'

Jacko nodded.

I pulled the towel off the cage to find Barney still pacing up and down the top perch. Jacko opened the door and picked the tin off the cage floor, then I reached through, towel in hand. It was a tight squeeze with three arms going through the little cage door. Jacko managed to tip the tin over Barney's head as I wrapped the towel about him. With much shrieking from the cockatoo, we eased him off his perch and out of the cage inside his towel cocoon. We'd only just got him out when the tin fell off, revealing a highly perturbed bird swinging his head from side to side, ready to bite anything he could reach.

I wasn't going to be able to hold the bird or fend off his beak for long. He was already starting to wiggle out of my grasp. I looked about the room.

'Jacko, grab one of those smaller cardboard boxes. That might be a safer place to hold him.'

Jacko pulled down a box and opened the lid, then I gently placed both bird and towel inside, swiftly closing the lid over the top. As sounds of scuffling and screaming pierced the cardboard, we heard Mavis call from the front, 'Is everything okay back there?'

'Yes, dear,' said Jacko at volume, while looking back to me with a lopsided grin.

As we regained our composure from our Barney-boxing experience, I pulled the mask off the end of the anaesthetic gas line. I'd decided to poke the tube straight into the box. It would take longer to take effect, but it was clearly going to be easier and safer all round than trying to put the mask on this bird. However, in order to complete my makeshift sedation chamber, I needed a bag to seal the box within to avoid Jacko and I also copping a dose of gas.

Jacko called out to Mavis, and within seconds a bag was passed though the door. I opened it up and placed the cardboard box into it, turning a deaf ear to the ongoing protest from inside, then wrapped the bag's opening tight around the gas hose and turned the anaesthetic machine on. I waited, checking every minute for continued sounds of movement until I was finally sure that Barney was asleep.

After instructing Jacko to hold his breath until any leftover gas dispersed, I opened up the box. Sure enough, the cockatoo was out of it. I replaced the mask onto to the end of the tube and placed it over Barney's face so as to continue feeding him the gas. He was still breathing well, and a quick check of his heart with my stethoscope revealed he was handling the anaesthetic well.

Now to work. I pulled out my nail clippers and trimmed his claws. That was the easy part done. Now to trim his beak and have a close inspection of that lump near his eye.

I turned to Jacko. 'I'll turn the gas off while I inspect his face. If you see him begin to move, let me know and I'll put it back on.'

Birds have an exceptionally fast metabolism, typically taking only seconds to awaken from anaesthesia, and I did not want to incur the wrath of Barney at very close quarters mid-procedure.

I opted to trim the beak first, thinking it better to reduce the length and sharpness of his main weapon as a first priority. He began to stir a little, so I snapped the mask back over his snout and gave him a few more breaths of anaesthetic. As I sat there I realised I could angle the mask so as to expose the eye while keeping his beak inside.

When I felt the lump, it was soft. I inserted a needle and drew out some yellow fluid, pus-like in appearance. I kept doing this until all the fluid had been drained, then administered an injection of pain relief and antibiotics into his breast muscle. He was quite plump under his plumage, with plenty of flesh in which to inject the medication.

After a quick check all over to ensure he was free of any other lumps, I turned off the anaesthetic while continuing the oxygen feed.

As I expected, Barney was awake again in less than a minute, and without a hint of doziness. Instead, he bore all the rage he'd carried with him before going under. He jumped back up before I had the chance to take hold of him, let alone get him back in his cage. With a defiant screech, he opened his wings and flew up onto the door frame.

I looked at Jacko. Jacko looked at me. *Here we go again.*

Jacko's gaze turned back to the box.

'If I can get the box over him, could you put the gas back on to at least quieten him down again?' he said.

I thought for a second, then nodded. I couldn't think of a better way to safely get him into the cage.

Jacko retrieved the box and with surprisingly little effort was able to trap Barney under it. As he did so, Barney's volume climbed again, and then someone tried to open the door from the other side.

'Don't come in!' we cried in unison.

A muffled voice offered an apology then retreated.

I inserted the hose though the bottom of the box and blasted the gas on. No time for plastic bags this time – I'd keep it short and sharp. Before long, we heard a distinct thump. I turned the gas off again, and Jacko whisked the box back towards the cage door. I picked up the bird's relaxed body and gently placed him on the floor of his enclosure, noticing a blink from one of his eyes as I completed the motion. By the time my hands were out of the cage and the door closed, he was back on his feet. He wobbled for just a moment before resuming his normal position on the top perch of the cage. With that he let out a stream of screeches clearly directed at Jacko and me. One could only imagine what the language would have been if it were translatable to English.

I opened the door into the shop and we wheeled the local celebrity back towards his rightful place out front. As we emerged from between the aisles, we were greeted by a round of applause. It turned out the small group of tourists I'd heard earlier had hung around over lunch and eavesdropped on the whole vet versus bird tussle. They had been well entertained.

Jacko and Mavis were very grateful for my efforts that day, but not Barney. He still greets me with a cursing squawk whenever I'm in town, while I keep all my digits and other body parts well clear of his cage. Perhaps I will go down in Tibooburra folklore as the only person who was ever able to touch Barney without being bitten.

DAWN'S FERAL CATS

The stench almost knocked me out. The odour of the urine of dozens of cats filled every corner of the shed. I had been warned by Dawn that there were quite a few cats, but nothing could have prepared me for this.

How does a woman come to have dozens of cats living in her backyard? You'd be surprised how easily it can happen. It starts with one – one feral cat you feel sorry for. You feed it, it comes back, you keep feeding it. Eventually it returns with a friend or two. Before long, some of those friends start having kittens. Cats are prolific breeders. They can have a litter every two months, especially in the cooler months, and they cycle while breastfeeding, so once the breeding starts, it can soon get out of hand. Before you know it, the one needy cat has become dozens of felines.

Every vet can list off the top of their heads the animal hoarders in their district. It's a common phenomenon, particularly with cats. Clowders – that's the collective noun for cats, in case you didn't know – of stray cats can be found on properties even in the middle of nowhere. There are many kind-hearted people like Dawn who don't realise what they are doing when they provide shelter to a stray cat, especially if they don't get the animal desexed. Cats, both domestic and feral, do serious damage to the wildlife population in both the bush and in urban environments in Australia. They don't need to be hungry to kill: they find entertainment in hunting birds and small marsupials and lizards.

Feline rescuers like Dawn don't intend to contribute to this damage. Cats are easy to love, at least for those of us who take to them, but unless they are carefully managed the highly evolved predator inside that purring ball of fluff is all too happy to reveal itself.

Dawn's first cat had been a little black female that started coming by in the evening. Within a few weeks, that cat had brought a couple of friends with her. Dawn opened her garden shed to them when they started having kittens, and she now found herself feeding 58 cats daily.

'I didn't want to harm them,' she tried to explain. After a phone call, I'd arranged to stop by on this road trip. She continued, 'I just wanted them to be safe.'

If I had a dollar for every time a cat rescuer has said that to me.

'But now there are so many!'

My eyes adjusted to the darkness within the small shed, the lights left off so as not to startle the animals. I could make out a mother cat with her kittens lying under some shelves in the far corner. Two other adult cats were lazing on the shelves above.

I edged towards them and squatted near the mother. The floor was covered in faeces, so I wasn't game to kneel if I could avoid it. She looked at me with some interest, her gaze lingering on the stethoscope about my neck. Animals always seem to have an innate ability to detect a vet within seconds of meeting us. Perhaps it's the underlying smell of antiseptic, like walking into a dental surgery.

I extended my hand towards the mother for a formal introduction. She tilted her head back, then pushed her nose forward to sniff my fingertips. She purred, which I took as acceptance of my attention. I gave her a few friendly strokes across her head and then along her back, while visually examining the kittens. There were six of them, three gingers and three grey. All looked healthy, about three weeks old, with their eyes open and just beginning to walk.

'I feed them all at night and, for those who want it, in the morning. I often lock them up for the night and then let them out in the morning. These are the friendlier ones that hang about the shed all day,' Dawn said, indicating the cats sitting around the shelving.

I stood up and looked her in the eye. Dawn was in her fifties, her long grey hair pulled into a neat bun.

'We need to come up with a plan,' I said. 'What would you like to happen to all the cats?'

'I'd like to rehome them, but I'm not sure if it's too late. Who would want an adult cat that's never been handled?'

I nodded. She was right. Rescue shelters are always overflowing with cats and kittens, and the unfortunate reality is that there are rarely enough people looking to give them a home. Cats that are unsuitable for rehoming are often euthanised as the only humane option.

I took a deep breath, the persistent odour almost causing me to gag.

'We have a few options. Let me lay them all out for you and you can decide how you feel comfortable with progressing.'

She nodded, solemn.

I continued. 'I can assess all the cats for temperament and health. There is a high chance that some will have FIV – feline AIDS – which can severely impact their quality of life as it weakens the immune system, similar to human AIDS. Any cats that test positive for FIV and are unhandled can be euthanised, or you can keep them aside and try to get them more friendly before trying to find them new homes. Putting these ones down is likely the more realistic option, as chances are slim that anyone is going to want to adopt an immunocompromised cat.'

It sounded brutal, but it was better than letting Dawn cherish false hope.

I continued. 'Cats that are healthy but so far unhandled can either be handled more to prepare them for potential rehoming, or we can put them down. Any cats that you want to rehome must be vaccinated, wormed and desexed.'

Dawn swallowed. 'That is going to be quite an expense.'

'Yes,' I said. 'Unfortunately, I'm not in a position where I'm able to do this for no cost. I don't receive any outside funding. You might be able to get the shire council to help out.'

'Will they put them down?' she asked.

I looked about the shed. In truth, the state in which these poor creatures were living was nothing short of appalling.

'They cannot continue to live like this,' I said, waving my arm to indicate the shed. 'And now that I am aware of this, I cannot leave them here in these conditions.'

I was hoping that Dawn would be coming to the realisation that she had to put the welfare of the cats above her emotional attachment to them.

One of the challenges of being a vet is that you find yourself caught between the conflicting interests of a person – your client – and an animal. It is my duty to place the welfare of animals first and foremost, though this can lead to difficult conversations when the human attached to the animal doesn't understand the condition the animal is living in or with. While I try to be as gentle as possible, I find myself lacking patience with the selfishness of some people and have little choice but to be blunt.

Dawn wasn't selfish, though I think she may have been in denial that she had a problem for some time. It had actually been her family who had contacted me, her daughters worried about their mum living with all these cats. Aside from the hygiene issues, they'd noticed that she was becoming reclusive. They'd given me a very detailed description of what to expect. Nevertheless, I had to get Dawn to agree for me to come. I'd rung her when I knew I would be in town during an upcoming road trip, telling her that I'd heard on the grapevine that she may have a cat problem, not telling her who had informed me. Thankfully it had been a productive conversation and she had been amenable to me coming around to visit and seeing if I had any suggestions about how to help her manage her cat population. Deep down I think she acknowledged that it was getting out of hand.

I waited with all the patience I could muster as Dawn looked about the shed, pondering her choices. I could see her grappling with her emotions as she came to terms with the reality of the situation.

After several minutes she relented. 'Okay, if you can assess them in the morning, I'll feed them all in the shed tonight and keep them in there.'

Later, I called the local council ranger to give him a heads up that he may find the pound inundated with cats the next day. Bob practically applauded me over the phone.

'I've been trying to get that lady to do something about those cats for months! I'll have the enclosures ready for them and bring over some carrier cages for transport.'

I was relieved. Some rangers refuse to help rehome cats. Ever since the New South Wales government brought in a law that domestic cats have the right to roam, it has made the job of managing the feral cat population extremely difficult for council animal officers.

The next morning, I met Dawn at the door of the shed. I'd heard the cacophony of meowing the minute I stepped out of my car.

From past experience, I was prepared for anything. There would be some timid cats and some aggressive ones. At least on this second visit I was more prepared for the smell, though it still violated my senses as we entered the shed together. Dawn slammed the door behind us to prevent any escapees as I located the light switch. With the room illuminated, I could see dozens of cats of mixed colours and ages. They all looked at us expectantly as it was past their breakfast time.

'I've counted them and they're all here. It's past their let-out time so they're extra noisy now.'

I sat my examination box on top of an old chest freezer in the corner. 'The ranger will be here soon. Have you decided which cats you'll keep?'

Dawn chewed on her lip. After a moment she had her answer. 'The mumma cat, the one under the shelves. That's the first cat who started coming around, so I'll keep her.'

I asked her to place that cat on the freezer for me to examine.

'I'll check her first, then the kittens. They're not ready to be weaned yet, so you'll need to keep them until then. They'll need vaccinations and worming once they're six weeks old. I'll give the mumma her vaccinations today.'

I liked this cat. Keeping her was a good decision. It would also give her time to raise the kittens, who would be much easier to rehome than the full-grown cats.

After I examined the little family and administered the mother's vaccine, Dawn placed them in a large cardboard box lined with a clean towel.

'I'll put them in my laundry,' she said.

As I opened the shed door for her, the ranger's car pulled into the drive. I stepped out behind Dawn and closed the door.

'G'day, Bob,' I said.

Bob was a short man with a large girth, his short black hair tucked under a ranger's wide-brimmed olive hat.

'G'day Doctor,' he said. He set about unloading cat cages from the back of the wagon. He had brought 20 cages with him, which would be enough to transport the cats to the pound.

I grabbed two cages in each hand and carried them to the shed. Dawn returned and between the three of us we built a tower of cages along the outside wall.

As we placed the last of the cages down, I turned to Bob and Dawn.

'Alright, here's the plan. We need to do this efficiently. Cats get stressed easily, so the less handling of the anxious ones, the better. Dawn, you pick each cat up and hold it in your arms while I examine it, then we'll place it into a cage. I'll pass the cage out the door to Bob as you pick up the next cat for me to examine.'

They both nodded.

I opened the shed and ushered Dawn in, and we got to work. Things went well. We didn't have enough cages for each cat to be held individually, so we doubled up on the first 30 or so that were reasonably easy to handle. Bob transferred these cages into his wagon.

'I haven't had much time with these ones,' said Dawn, indicating the remaining animals, mostly large tomcats. Many of them bore scars, some fresh, from fighting each other over females and territory. These ones weren't going to be easy. As anyone who's handled a cantankerous cat knows, once a cat has decided it doesn't want to be held, there is no talking them around. Cats that have had minimal human contact are especially feisty. Dawn coaxed a few out and I was able to give them a very brief examination before depositing them into a carrier. These ones were extremely timid due to their lack of handling, but they hadn't been aggressive, so there was hope that they could be adopted out.

That left ten large, older male toms, all straight out of 'angry cat' central casting. Each had allocated itself a corner or high vantage point on a shelf, and as we tried to approach, they were all arched backs, bared teeth, exposed claws and spiteful hisses. I looked at Dawn after we had tried, without success, to coax a few of them to us. There was a large ginger male sitting on a shelf at about my eye height. I thought he seemed the least aggressive out of the boys. I approached him slowly, while he stared at me with a mix of curiosity and restrained anger. As I reached out my hand in a peace offering, he remained still. I extended my fingers for him to sniff and held my breath. He didn't move towards my hand, so I reached a little further, at which the hair on his back stood up and he began a low growl. I froze. He continued to growl. *You win*, I thought, taking a step back and lowering my arm.

I looked back at Dawn and shrugged. 'I don't know if we're going to get anywhere with these guys.'

'I'm afraid these are likely beyond rehoming,' Dawn admitted, taking the words out of my mouth.

'No, I don't see them becoming family pets in a hurry,' I said.

She sighed dejectedly, knowing that the tough call had to be made. I put a hand on her arm, comforting her as she found the courage to permit me to do what had to be done.

'Alright. Well, I can't keep them,' she said. 'They're only going to keep fighting each other.'

'I'll give them a quick, painless end,' I assured her. I hated that this waste of life had to happen, especially as it could easily have been prevented if they'd been desexed earlier.

'How are we going to catch them?' Dawn asked.

'I'll ask Bob if he has a cat trap I can borrow.'

Outside, Bob was loading the last of the tame cats into the wagon. He handed me a medium-sized trap.

'That's done the trick for me many times,' he said. 'Do you need some help in there?'

'Thank you, Bob. That would be appreciated.'

With Bob's assistance, I could spare Dawn the pain of being involved in this next step. She had a look of horror on her face when she saw the cat trap.

'I know it looks barbaric, but it's the safest way to handle them for what we have to do,' I said. I explained that I would give them a sedation so that they wouldn't feel any pain, then administer the euthanasia drug, which is a type of anaesthetic. 'I'm basically deliberately giving them an overdose of anaesthetic. They will go into a deep sleep that they won't awaken from.'

'I'll be outside if you don't mind,' she said softly.

Bob held the cage open near the first cat as I used a towel to encourage it inside, feeling like a matador. My 'bull' might have been very small, but what it lacked in size it made up for in venomous anger. I was as careful as possible to avoid the claws and teeth. I sedated, then euthanised the cat. Then we repeated the process. After about 30 minutes we had completed the horrendous task. Bob offered to take the euthanised cats with him and bury them in the council's pet cemetery.

I've had colleagues who've been severely emotionally impacted by having to carry out this sort of mass euthanasia. It's so draining, even when we know it is the most humane option, and really the only option for animals that have no hope of being rehomed. Sadly, thousands of unwanted animals get put down by vets every day.

I emerged from the shed that day emotionally wrecked and annoyed at the whole scenario. This problem of feral and stray cats could be rectified, or at least mitigated, by a government-funded, community-driven program to desex domestic cats before they reach breeding age. This would allow vets, rangers and shelters to manage feral populations in a kinder manner, with less need for mass culling.

I didn't blame Dawn. She was a good person who'd thought she was doing the right thing when she'd taken in the first and subsequent cats. I could also see that she was as upset as I was by the morning's activities. Still, as we packed up to leave, she was already coming to accept that it had all been necessary.

'I'll drop by in about a month, on my next run through town, to vaccinate the kittens,' I said. 'I'll also be able to desex mum then.'

When I returned a month later, I hardly recognised Dawn. She was much brighter, without as much of the weight of the world on her shoulders, now that she only had a small number of cats to care for. 'Now I'm not embarrassed to have visitors into my home,' she told me. She'd been socialising again and her family were more willing to visit. The cats she'd saved were in good shape too, and Dawn was pleased to tell me that she'd already found homes for all the little ones.

'I'm not surprised,' I said. 'It's always much easier to find homes for cute little kittens like this. But do make sure you tell the new owners to have them desexed at six months.'

Dawn nodded as I handed her the signed vaccination certificates.

'Hopefully I don't need to see you for a while,' she said. 'No offense.'

'None taken,' I replied, shaking her hand.

None of this had been ideal, but at least we'd been able to give most of the adult cats good homes, and certainly much better lives than they could have expected fending for themselves in the wild.

PREG TESTING WHILE PREGNANT

The plane bumped about, the April day unseasonably hot with strong northerly winds lifting the dust into a storm. Not the best flying conditions, especially in my condition. I was pregnant, Brendan and I having received the happy confirmation of this state of affairs about five months earlier. The stifling atmosphere in the cabin wasn't helped by the fact that my aeroplane has no air conditioning. I rely on keeping the vents open to provide some cooler air, but dust and open vents don't go well together.

I grimaced as I checked my maps, ensuring I was still on course. It's difficult to navigate in the outback at the best of times, given how few landmarks there are to aid you in navigation. During dry spells, as this country near the New South Wales–South Australia border was still going through at the time, everything blurs into one. While I could see some patches of dry feed, there were vast spans of bare, thirsty earth below. No wonder the soil was being lifted by the wind. My eyes rarely left the compass as I kept the aircraft locked on its heading. Eventually, making out a road beneath me and cross-referencing my charts, I worked out I was only 20 nautical miles from the station airstrip, so I switched my UHF to their channel.

'Calling Burr Creek, anyone on channel?'

Hannah's voice crackled across the radio. 'I'm here, waiting on the southern end. There's a bloody strong northerly down here.'

I allowed myself a smile. It's always good to have someone on the ground who understands a pilot's needs and can provide you with an accurate wind direction at ground level. Parking her car at the southern end of the strip, safely to the side, would help me identify my landing point.

'No dramas, Hannah. I'll set up to land into the breeze.'

When my GPS indicated that I was within 10 nautical miles of the station, I set up for landing by lowering the landing gear and checking the oil pressure. I gave the rudder pedals a push to ensure my brakes were working and that the wheels were locked down. Giving the plane a rough jolt with the rudder helped reassure me that all was in order.

Through the rusty haze of the dust storm I could make out a white ute in front of my bird's nose, and as I got closer I could see the outline of the airstrip. Pockets of turbulence buffered the plane as I got closer to the ground, but I ignored them, concentrating on landing. Landing a plane always requires your full attention, even more so in more trying conditions. I reduced power, set full flaps and, just above the ground, pulled back on the controls to lift my nose before the wheels skidded onto the surface.

I parked halfway along the airstrip, nose pointed into the wind, then lumbered myself and my swollen belly out of the cockpit. I pulled out the tie-down ropes and cover as Hannah pulled up beside me.

'Lovely day for it,' I called out over the wind as she trudged towards me holding her Akubra on her head. The hat's top was punched up, which is the customary fashion for folks in this corner of the district.

We shook hands and I started hammering in the first peg.

'Here, I'll tie for you,' she offered.

Hannah was a small woman in her late fifties, standing about 5 foot 6 (168cm). She grew up with my father and so we knew each other well. She was a lady of the land, the lines across her tanned face a testament to the hard work she had done. Her blonde hair was tucked into a bun at the base of her neck, underneath the weather-beaten hat.

I passed her the ropes, then continuing hammering. I only needed to hammer in three pegs, one for each wing and another for the tail, but the ground was hard. After years of rolling, the strip was well compacted. It took multiple smacks with the hammer and more than a few curse words before I got the pegs down. Hannah attached the ropes to the plane using the tie points located under each wing and tail. After double-checking them, the two of us pulled the cover over the aircraft and clipped it down over the windows. Hannah's help was appreciated again. In this wind, the cover could easily have been whisked away from me.

Jobs done, we retreated to the shelter of the ute's cabin. My job today was to do pregnancy tests on Hannah's nephew Steve's cattle on the adjacent property, so she would drive me the 40-minute trip over there. It would be a 'quick job', I was told. How many times have I heard that before?

'It's only a few hundred head of cows. We've got good new yards and a strong crush,' Steve had told me on the phone. He reassured me that it would be safe for me. In theory my work should only take a couple of hours, so if I flew over at midday and did the cows just after they'd been yarded, I would have plenty of time to get home before dark.

'How's the muster going?' I asked Hannah.

'The boys are getting a bit of a pizzling out there today,' she said, using a local term for having a tough time of it. 'They should be in the yards by the time we get there.'

The 'boys' were all grown men in their thirties now, but they would always be boys to Hannah.

Hannah leaned forward and turned up the UHF. Instantly the radio blared with the voices of the men.

'Yeah, this one's not playing the game. She keeps trying to knock me off the bike,' said someone who I thought might be Steve.

'Leave it,' replied Russ. Russ had a new, small aircraft and was now the chief mustering pilot in the family business.

Hannah and I shared a smirk. They were getting a pizzling.

I picked up the handset. 'G'day Russ, I've landed. Hannah and I are on our way over.'

'No worries, Ameliah. We're a few kilometres from the yards but should be close by the time you get there,' Russ replied.

That sounded optimistic to me. I started feeling a bit uneasy about the whole thing. If the cattle weren't in the yards by the time we got there, there wasn't much chance I would get the job done in time to fly home today.

Mustering on large properties is a major exercise. Essentially, it means rounding up all the animals – cattle, sheep, or goats on our place – in a very large paddock. The beasts can be spread out over several kilometres when we start, so first we have to find them all. That's where aircraft, either fixed-wing or helicopters, really earn their keep. Pilots can get people on the ground where the animals are. With skilful flying close to the ground, they can also start the herding process before others on motorbikes or horses, often aided by well-trained dogs, gradually bring the mob together then funnel them, sometimes over several kilometres, towards the yards.

Being a passenger on a mustering flight is a good test of your stomach, as the aircraft whoops and dives and turns on a point on an invisible and seemingly endless roller coaster of air. That said, today's flights sound tame compared with the reputed antics of my grandfather. In the days before UHF radio was available for communication, he would place a hand-drawn mud-map showing the location of animals into a glass bottle, then drop the bottle out the plane for the men on the ground to collect. Their job at that point was to stay clear of falling glass. The story goes that the bottles never broke.

We were planning a muster at our place the next day. It's usually a family affair. Until (and if) he passes the pilot's role to me, Dad flies in his Cessna while Brendan and I ride motorbikes; Sue provides home support. Occasionally we employ one or two others to assist. If it's goats we're chasing, we hire a contractor, Dwayne, and his team of Indigenous lads. Goats are particularly difficult to muster. It's not unusual to have a mob of a hundred goats together when pushing them through a patch of dense scrub, only to have just half a dozen pop out the other side. Dwayne and the boys do a great job, with plenty of humour in the mix. That's useful, because the atmosphere can get a bit tense during mustering, with any small misunderstanding often leading to escaped animals and wasted time. Brendan and I try to adhere to a rule that what happens in the paddock stays in the paddock, though there are definitely times when each of us feels like leaving the other out there.

Back at Steve's place, Hannah and I continued listening to the boys' banter as we made our way northwards through several 10,000-acre paddocks, past fences built for cattle with five rows of straight wire and a line of barbed wire along the top to deter any hurdlers. The thermometer on the car's dash read 36°C as the outside temperature. However, Hannah had plenty of cool water on board and an esky filled with delicious goodies to nibble on. I remembered the lecture Brendan had given me that morning about looking after myself, so I took advantage of what Hannah had on offer.

As we approached the yards, I could see they sat empty. Beyond them, still some distance away through the scrub, a telltale cloud of dust signalled the location of the mob. While it was perfectly comfortable sitting in the ute with Hannah, enjoying the cool and shelter, I couldn't help the nagging feeling that it was going to be a long afternoon.

Over the radio we heard Russ tell the team that he was going to call it a day and land his plane.

'What's the wind like down there, Hannah?' he asked.

Hannah looked to me, eyebrows raised. Was he planning to land at the yards? The hopbush in the scrub was being buffeted sideways by the wind.

'The forecast was for 40-knot northerly winds at 2000 feet. Judging by the trees down here, I'd say it's about the same on the ground,' said Hannah.

There was a brief silence over the radio before Russ said, 'That sounds like too much crosswind for me. I'll go back and land at the airstrip and drive back.'

An expression of relief washed over Hannah's face.

Within minutes, the herd of cattle and three following motorbikes emerged from the bushes, moving towards the wing of the yards. Hannah and I left the ute and walked through the yards, making certain all the gates were open to accept the herd, then returned to the cabin to keep out of the way. The cacophony of mooing cattle and revving motorbikes grew to a crescendo as the mob approached, as did the cloud of dust. Finally all the animals were herded into the yard, the bike riders parking behind the gates once they were latched closed.

As the three men walked towards the ute, Hannah and I got out and pulled cold drinks from the esky. Steve, Brayden and Junada accepted these gratefully as I shook hands with each of them. All bore the hallmarks of the day's work so far, dust over tanned faces and through their dark hair.

'Well, things could have gone worse,' said Steve dryly.

Brayden rolled his eyes. 'I don't know how it could get any worse.' His can of lemonade was already empty, crushed and thrown into the back of the ute before he finished speaking. The other blokes soon followed suit.

As I picked up my box of gloves and wandered over to the yards, Steve and Brayden went to a trailer and lifted out a set of cattle scales. I groaned inwardly. I hadn't banked on the cattle being weighed. It's a tedious task and I would have to wait for each cow's weight to register before I could step in behind them to do pregnancy diagnosis. On top of the late start, this 'quick job' was going to take a lot longer than anticipated.

Brayden turned to me. 'Don't get too enthusiastic yet. It'll take a bit for us to set the scales up before you can start.'

I nodded and put the box of gloves down outside of the yards, my heart sinking a little further.

It took a fair bit of improvising to set the scales into the dirt floor of the crush. The boys put down a piece of corrugated iron to create a level surface on which to sit them, then used a few lengths of wire to fix the scales to that floor. It wasn't the concrete base the scales were designed for, but it would have to do.

I checked that the kick gate, which would stop any animal launching a stray hoof at me, was still able to close properly with the scales in place. With Brendan's concerns ringing in my ears, I was determined to be extra cautious, double-checking that each cow was firmly caught in the head bail of the crush and that the kick gate was safely secure.

'Right, let's get you some cows,' Brayden said, sprinting down the race to start pushing the cattle up.

Finally I pulled my gloves on, more than two hours after I'd landed at Hannah's place. Time was ticking on apace, but sadly the cattle didn't share my urgency. Pregnancy testing is a messy job. You're literally up to your armpits in cow shit, your arm inserted deep into the cow's rectum to the point where you can feel the uterus underneath. I yell 'empty' when there's a small muscular uterus and 'pregnant' when the uterus is fluid-filled or I can feel a developed calf foetus, with its leg or nose greeting my fingertips. Thanks to all the practice I'd had back on the

Archard's property outside Kerang, I'd become quite quick at the procedure. I can usually do close to a hundred cows an hour through a good crush with plenty of helpers keeping the cattle flowing along. In this case it took an hour to get through the first forty cows.

The scales kept misreading as they got bumped about in the bottom of the crush. Meanwhile the cattle, fresh out of the paddock, were still jumpy and easily stirred, so just feeding them along the race was slower. If there was a plus, it was that by the time they were weighed they'd settled a little in the crush before I got behind them, but I did spend a lot of time twiddling my gloved thumbs between tests. As they always do, each cow jolted about when I inserted my arm into her backside – I guess this is understandable – but the crush and gates ensured that my own unborn child was kept safe through the process.

We had worked though half the mob when a wagon drove up to the yards. Out climbed a bunch of kids, as well as Steve and Brayden's wives, Michelle and Tania, and a couple of containers of sandwiches. Steve turned up in his vehicle soon afterwards. Time for a break and some tucker to recharge.

One of the young boys begged Steve, 'Dad, can I push the cows up the race?'

Steve and his wife Michelle shared a look, then Steve put a hand on his son's shoulder. 'Probably not safe for you to be in the yards with this lot, mate. When we're finished, you can help me take them out on your motorbike.'

The boy chewed his lip and then nodded, satisfied with this plan.

Michelle began packing up the lunch. 'I'll give you a hand if Tania doesn't mind watching the kids,' she said.

Tania was happy with this plan and took up a position on the edge of Hannah's ute tray, her baby in her arms. The rest of us resumed our positions, Michelle helping to keep the feed of cattle flowing. The job progressed as fast as it could, given the haphazard setup, though several times the wire twitches holding the scales in place had to be replaced, causing further hold ups. By now I was resigned to not being able to get away before dark, watching the sun sink further towards the horizon as the afternoon got away from us.

As we paused for yet another broken twitch, I excused myself to make a phone call. We were going to be mustering ourselves the next day, which added to my disappointment at not being able to get home as planned.

When Brendan didn't answer, I rang Dad.

'No dramas,' said Dad when I told him the story. 'We can start the muster with a smaller paddock. Brendan and I can handle the job.'

Returning to the yards, I confirmed I was good to hang around until we'd done the whole herd.

'I knew Bluey would cope,' said Steve, clapping me on the back.

I returned a half-hearted smile. As much as I enjoyed their company, much like a rabbit I would have much preferred to be sleeping in my own hutch.

'Who else would you rather be working with?' joked Russ.

'Maybe don't answer that,' said Steve before I could respond.

'At least you get to spend the night with Hannah and old Trev,' said Brayden.

I smiled at that. I hadn't seen Trev for a while, and I always found his stories of the old times interesting. And I had to admit to myself that flying home first thing in the morning would be far more pleasant than bracing the dust-laden skies again this evening.

The sun hung low in the sky as we finished. Despite the slow pace of the job, we had all emerged without any serious injuries. Brayden had jammed his hand in the crush, but only had grazes on the back of his hand to show for it.

'I reckon you've all earned one of these,' said Hannah, delving into her esky again and passing around cold cans of beer. As she thoughtfully handed me a lemonade, I wondered ruefully whether a beer would be more dangerous to my child than spending an afternoon working with fiery cattle.

We stood around the back of the ute, swapping yarns as the sun set. I enjoyed listening as I drank the cold, bubbly drink, feeling my energy levels recharging with every sip.

Steve's son was soon at his father to get going so that he could help take the cattle out.

'Okay, okay,' he relented finally. The kids piled into the old four-wheel-drive wagon.

'Thanks for coming,' said Brayden, before he and the rest of the crew went to let the cattle out.

Hannah and I watched the cattle trot out of the yards, pausing on the flat, bare area before the bushes. Steve drove the wagon up and down the edge of the scrub, holding them up so that they would settle down and wander back to their pasture in a sensible manner.

I took a few minutes to admire the sight before me. It's rare to see such a large gathering of family working in unison. This particular family have achieved much over the years. Each couple had their own property that they lived on and managed, but they all pitched in together on the more labour-intensive jobs, rarely needing to hire contractors. The organisation can be haphazard, but it seems to work well.

I spent a pleasant night at the homestead, Hannah making dinner while Trev shared a few tales. While I'd have loved to be at home, if I had to be held up somewhere, this was the place to be. Good food and good company. What more could you wish for in life?

CLOSING A CIRCLE

It was eight o'clock on a Friday night in late winter. Brendan was watching the AFL and I was reading a book when a gentle double kick from the little being inside me broke my waters.

'Right, everything in the car. Now!'

Brendan looked up in disbelief, a block of chocolate poised halfway to his mouth. This wasn't the plan. I was booked in for a caesarean section the next week and we had intended to drive to Broken Hill the next day to wait out the remaining time. Seems our baby had other ideas.

Brendan dropped the chocolate and grabbed my pile of hospital-ready items from the front door, throwing them into the back of our ute. He then returned to the bedroom, grabbed an overnight bag and started to chuck clothes into it.

You've got to be kidding, I thought to myself. He'd seen my bag packed at the front door for weeks, but chose to wait until now to pack a bag for himself? I would have doubled over with laughter at the situation if I'd been able to.

I called the nearest hospital, 80 kilometres away in Wilcannia, and let them know we were on our way in. We drove there at a reasonable pace; it was too dangerous to go fast. We dodged various kangaroos and potholes along the way. By the time we got there my contractions were six minutes apart. Wilcannia is only a very small health service, so they had arranged for the Royal Flying Doctor Service (RFDS) to meet us and transfer me to Broken Hill. Brendan would follow in the car.

During the flight, my labour really kicked in. The contractions ramped up as we left the tarmac, and by the time we got to Broken Hill they were only two minutes apart. The flight nurse high-fived me as we landed, happy that they'd got me there in one piece. I was wheeled straight into theatre, and just after midnight our little bundle of joy arrived. Brendan got there just as she was being placed into my arms. He might have made it for the birth itself if he hadn't needed to fill up his perpetually empty fuel tank on the way.

We later dropped off a carton of cider to the RFDS crew who had been on duty that night. For those of us who live in remote Australia, it is difficult to put a value on this service on which we know we can rely.

We named our daughter Lindsay, after the man who'd sold me his aeroplane, and started to come to terms with the enormous impact this little bundle would have on our lives.

Like all parents, we completely underestimated the level of disruption a newborn would bring, but we got to work making adjustments to fit her in. In particular, I couldn't just throw my vet bag into the plane and take off to a job on the spur of the moment anymore. Instead, I made all my appointments pre-booked so that I could organise someone to look after Lindsay. Often that was Brendan, but sometimes I needed to look further afield. Over time, Brendan took on more of the parenting load to allow me to restart my road trips too.

Between being a mother, a vet and a farmer, I also needed to make sure that I had some time for myself. We worked out that the best time for that was an hour before dawn, when I could spend time outside with my own animals, taking the dogs for a walk or putting a horse through its paces. Sometimes I could get in a ride in the evening too, just as the sun was setting. On the best days, when the lake isn't completely full, its sandy shores became my equine arena. A light breeze across the water and through the gum trees as the day cools makes it the most magical experience. A brief moment for reflection and solitude.

Early one morning in late 2021, I found myself back where I had started: sitting next to Dad in his Cessna.

I'd been up early to prepare my own plane for a flight to a station west of us, about an hour away by air. However, after powering up I discovered a problem with the Arrow's constant speed propeller. It was likely a cable problem and easily fixed, but I had an appointment to keep and no time to mess around with it. I looked across the hangar at Dad's Cessna 172 sitting beside the avgas bowser. *She'll have to do*, I thought, as I shut the engine of the Arrow down. I did a check over the Cessna, including ensuring she had enough fuel onboard, then raced over to the main house, where I knew Dad would still be enjoying his morning coffee.

'My plane is a no-go this morning. Could I take yours?' I said, adding, 'and could you come?'

It had been over a year since I'd flown this plane, so I felt a little rusty. Plus I still didn't really feel comfortable taking his pride and joy without him.

Ever the good bloke, Dad agreed to join me for this little adventure. It was a short trip to do still more pregnancy testing of cows. I had to be back by lunchtime as I had a little baby to breastfeed. I'd already risen an hour before dawn to give Lindsay a big drink before preparing for my flight. Yes, you can be a mother and a flying vet; it just takes a lot more preparation.

Dad and I prepared his plane and took to the air, flying in a similar direction to the one I'd been heading when I visited Hannah's place; that is, west, towards the South Australian border. Shaun's station was past Packsaddle, and I'd already texted him to tell him that I was running late.

It was the beginning of summer and the heat had already burnt off what little greenery there was. From 2000 feet up, the landscape looked mostly red, with brown patches indicating open grass flats. The further we travelled west, the more arid the land became. With the drought not having properly broken, properties like Shaun's were in 'limp' mode, the feed in the paddocks enough to keep stock alive, but little more. It was a stark contrast to the thriving season we were having at home.

I spotted the cattle yards as we approached our destination, and the airstrip soon became visible to the south, parallel to the road. I pulled the throttle out to slow us down and set up for landing. Having not flown this girl for a while, I was a little high in my approach, so I pulled the throttle out further still as well as pulling on full flaps to drag us back a few more knots in speed. The 172 floated a little along the runway as we came in to land, as these high-wings often do, but I softly connected the wheels to the ground. I gave Dad a satisfied smile, pleased that I still had my aviation touch as I parked on the end of the red runway.

Shaun met us in his four-wheel-drive wagon. In his mid-forties, he was considered a young bloke in these parts. With a fair complexion and sandy hair, he stood about six feet (183cm) tall. Between him and Dad, I felt very short.

I shook his hand, explaining why we were late and why Dad was with me.

'How're you goin', Blue? It's been a while since I've seen you.'

'Good to see you too, mate,' said Dad. 'I thought I'd better come and see if I can earn myself a living as a vet's assistant. How much do you reckon I'll get paid?'

I scoffed. 'Probably the same amount that I get paid as a station hand.'

Shaun drove us to the yards, where there were about 400

cattle waiting. All were the dark-brown, large-framed northern cattle of the Santa Gertrudis breed.

There were no helpers to be seen.

'Leave for two seconds and the staff think they're on holidays,' Shaun grumbled. 'Give me a minute to round up the troops.' He picked up the UHF radio handset.

I was pleased to know that we did have some manpower for the job.

A couple of minutes later a cloud of dust rose up as a vehicle raced towards the yards. Two strapping young blokes hopped out.

'We just had to get my phone,' one explained.

'It's not essential to have your phone on you for this job, is it?' said Shaun.

'He might miss out on a Tinder match,' I said, giving the young bloke a wink.

With that, we entered the yards and began to push the cattle up towards the crush. I donned my gloves, ready for work. Dad positioned himself in the forcing yard at the back of the race. It's not the best spot for an older fella to be, as it can be dangerous if a fiery beast decides to take you on. It's even less sensible when you're wearing a new prosthetic leg, long overdue thanks to COVID delays. However, I said nothing. I'm always being told off by Dad for being bossy, so this time I figured I'd keep my mouth shut.

The other young blokes positioned themselves along the race to keep the cattle flowing up to me, while Shaun manned the head bail that would catch each one and hold it to ensure my safety as I conducted my work. The day started well, the cattle flowing nicely … until a few temperamental girls created havoc.

'Look out!' someone yelled.

I turned to see Dad clambering up the rails to get away from an angry cow. He got to the top just in time, as she pulled up underneath his feet. She snorted at his shadow, stomping the ground. Dad stayed put as we started again.

Then Shaun missed catching a particularly fast cow as it raced through the crush.

'Bugger, that's a carton I owe,' he said.

In the farming world, beer is the currency that pays for mistakes. The usual penalty for letting a cow through the crush is a slab of beer.

'We'll try to get her back in,' Shaun said as he opened the gate into the forcing yard. With that, the fiery cow rushed out to join her escapee friend, the two cows now jogging around the middle work yard. I took refuge inside the crush as they ran past.

The men tried for several minutes to encourage the cows back into the forcing yard, keeping close to the rails as they did so. The cows tried to charge at them on several occasions. Finally, though, they moved to where they were supposed to be and the gate was slammed closed behind them.

'Right, back to it,' said Shaun.

We continued with the other cows, who had been waiting patiently in the race.

'Look out, Blue!' one of the young blokes shouted again.

I turned around to see Dad's nemesis rearing up the rails at him again. He sat precariously planted upon the top rail while she rubbed her head against the rails and his good leg, before tossing her head up and knocking Dad off his seat. He fell backwards towards the ground, head first. His cigarettes flew from his pocket, followed by his spectacles and hat, before he came to earth with a cringeworthy thump.

We raced over as he collected himself.

'I'm fine, I'm fine. Just let me get my smokes,' he said as replaced his hat on his head.

He picked up his cancer sticks, but didn't argue with this doctor's orders to sit down in the shade, drink some water and swallow some Panadol. As we continued with the job at hand, I noted that he wasn't sucking through his cigarettes at his usual pace, a sure sign that he must have been feeling below average. You can't tell these old fellas. They've got to learn for themselves when it's time to get out of the bloody road. There were plenty of young, agile people on this job who could have been in the forcing yard instead of him.

Finally, the job was done. To Shaun's delight, there were only a handful of empty cows. I pulled off my gloves, revealing my prune-like fingers. The sweat that had built up inside the gloves had treated my fingers like a swimming pool. I excused myself to go change into a clean set of clothes behind one of the cars. The blokes, respecting my privacy, made small talk at the crush side, before leaving the yards once I emerged re-dressed.

I offered Dad a swig of my cold water bottle before I guzzled most of it down. I noticed he had a small graze along the side of his face, but I said nothing. I'd wait until we were imprisoned in the plane to have that chat. I thought about how the roles of fathers and daughters change over time. As my father gets older, I sometimes feel that I'm the parent now, giving lectures on safety that he ignores.

As it turned out, I didn't need to say much. As we flew back towards home, I asked how he was going. He admitted that his pride was the most hurt.

'I thought I was a young fella again,' he admitted.

'Yes, well. There are plenty of young blokes around, so you don't need to be putting yourself in those situations,' I said.

'We won't be telling Sue about this,' he said.

'Best not,' I agreed.

As we circled home in preparation for landing, I couldn't help thinking about how far I'd come since that flight with Dad to Amanda's place a few years earlier, my very first, if unofficial, job as a flying vet. Since then, I'd accrued my own aeroplane, a husband and a daughter. I'd set up and equipped my own practice, with a growing list of clients spread between the Queensland and Victorian borders, and we were now living on my favourite piece of this planet. I had no desire to be anywhere else.

There are plenty more adventures to come. There'll come a day when Lindsay and her brother James (born as I was penning the final words to this book) will start to make their own ways in the world, and may or may not want to stay out here, but that day is a long way off. For now I'm enjoying the experience of being a wife, mother and farmer, while continuing to live my dream of being a flying vet.

ACKNOWLEDGEMENTS

To Simone Landes from The Lifestyle Suite, a remarkable woman without whom the opportunity to write this book would not have happened.

To the team at HarperCollins for their dedication on this project.

And to David Brewster for his help in writing this book.